Paul A. Byrne
Defender of Life

Christopher W. Bogosh

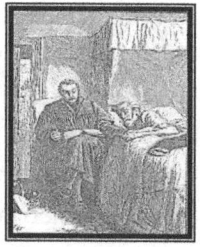

Good Samaritan Books

Paul A. Byrne: Defender of Life
Copyright © 2024 Christopher W. Bogosh
Published by Good Samaritan Books
        86395 Riverwood Drive
        Yulee, FL 32097
        goodsamaritanbooks@gmail.com

All rights reserved. No part of this publication may be reproduced, stored in a retrieval system, or transmitted in any form by any means, electronic, mechanical, photocopy, recording, or otherwise, without the publisher's prior permission, except as provided by the United States of America copyright law.

Printed in the United States of America
ISBN: 9798884725492

Dedicated

To the late Dr. John Schweiss (1925-2012), who taught Dr. Byrne, "As long as the person is alive, you have to keep trying to figure out what to do until the person dies."

Contents

Author's Preface

Introduction: Dr. Paul Byrne
~1~

1

Protector and Defender of Joseph
~21~

2

"Brain Death — An Opposing Viewpoint"
~55~

3

"Declaration of Death Requires Understanding Life"
~95~

4

"The Uniform Determination of Death Act (UDDA):
Repeal and Replace"
~159~

Author's Preface

In 2014, I had my first correspondence with Dr. Byrne. I was working on *Modern Medicine's Definition of Death: Ethical Implications for Christians*, and he reviewed parts of it. At the time, I didn't agree with some of his criticisms. My disagreements stemmed from views about death I developed while working as a hospice nurse, but some of these have changed thanks to Dr. Byrne.

I was more focused on palliative care to treat symptoms rather than aggressive care to prolong life. While there is a delicate balance and overlap between the two approaches to these treatment strategies, the Bible is clear, death is an enemy, and we should hope for and pursue its destruction (1 Cor. 15:26).

In the United States (US), we have developed a cozy friendship with death, at least when it comes to other people's deaths. Such is the case when harvesting organs from non-responsive organ donors and implanting them in other people deemed more worthy to live. The cause of death for organ donors declared dead under US law today is the removal of their organs, and this is primarily what *Paul A. Byrne: Defender of Life* is about.

Throughout the past few years, I've had the honor and privilege to meet and become intimately acquainted with Dr. Byrne. As the reader will see, he is a delightful person, a devout follower of Jesus, and absolutely brilliant. Alongside all of this is a tireless zeal to oppose "brain death" as death and to protect vulnerable people. I was truly blessed by researching and writing about his life. I am humbled by Dr. Byrne's willingness to trust me to put it all together.

Christopher W. Bogosh
Season of Resurrection, 2024
Yulee, Florida

Introduction: Dr. Paul Byrne

Dr. Paul Byrne was born on St. Valentinus Day in *Anno Domini* (AD) 1933, or February 14, Valentine's Day, to Randolph and Anna Byrne at the height of the Great Depression in Norwood, "The Gem of the Highlands," a city surrounded by Cincinnati, Ohio. Dr. Byrne is a third-generation Irish-German immigrant.

After Dr. Byrne's parents married, they settled in Norwood, a small frontier community established in 1870 with a population of fewer than 500 pioneers. The Marietta & Cincinnati Railroad arrived in 1875, only twenty-five years before the births of Dr. Byrne's parents. Dr. Byrne's father worked as a residential builder in the frontier boomtown, and his mother was a housewife.

In 1902, Cincinnati attempted to annex Norwood. However, the then 6,000-plus citizens voted to incorporate their town into a city, preventing the annexation. Norwood was now a burgeoning city with economic prosperity, but that was before the Great Depression. "My father owned more than one house," Dr. Byrne recalled. However, the city's real lifeline lay not in capitalist greed but in the devotion of its citizens to Roman Catholicism, traditional family values, and a hard work ethic.

Construction of Mount St. Mary's Seminary was completed ten years before Dr. Byrne was born. It was the faithful zeal of Roman Catholic clergy to administer grace to Norwood's residents that gave faith, hope, and diligent perseverance amidst adversity. All three factors, devotion to Jesus Christ, the Great Depression, and Dr. Byrne's birth on Valentine's Day, would impact his life, calling, and destiny as a pro-life medical doctor.

As noted above, at one time, Valentine's Day was associated with St. Valentinus, a third-century martyr who ministered to persecuted Christians when Claudius II Gothicus was Emperor of the Roman World. During the high Middle Ages, St. Valentinus's Day became associated with courtly love, and it passed into modern times with romantic overtones.

Valentine's Day has since been associated with National Donor Day. According to the website promoting the annual event: "National Donor Day is a time to focus on all types of donations" by appealing to the spirit of charity to inspire organ, tissue, and blood donation. In 1933, the world was oblivious to what would become a multibillion-dollar transplant business. Nevertheless, Dr. Byrne's love for vulnerable human beings and his defense of them would be stirred later in life by the spirit of St. Valentinus.

While organ transplant surgeries were still a dream of the future in 1933, the people in the United States (US) were aware of the realities of the Great Depression. In the US, the Great Depression was linked to the stock market crash on "Black Thursday," October 24, 1929, under President Herbert Hoover's administration. By the time Franklin Delano Roosevelt (FDR) was inaugurated president on March 4, 1933, the banking system had collapsed, roughly 25 percent of the labor force was unemployed, and economic prosperity had fallen dramatically.

According to the National Archives:

Reduced prices and reduced output resulted in lower incomes in wages, rents, dividends, and profits throughout the economy. Factories were shut down, farms and homes were lost to foreclosure, mills and mines were abandoned, and people went hungry. The resulting lower incomes meant the further inability of the people to spend or to save their way out of the crisis, thus perpetuating the economic slowdown in a seemingly never-ending cycle.

Dr. Byrne entered the world in this time and space, and the situation profoundly impacted his outlook on life and selfless spirit.

During the Great Depression, "My parents lost everything," Dr. Byrne recalled. "Since nothing was being built, my father was happy to get any job, as were my uncles. If any of them got a job for a day's pay, they bought food, rationed it, and shared it." Dr. Byrne continued: "My parents only completed the eighth grade. We never had much money, even after the Great Depression. I didn't have a bicycle until I was about ten years old. After FDR's new program was set into motion, my father no longer worked as a builder but got a job as a fireman."

"Eventually," Dr. Byrne recalled, "my father became a Fire Inspector, and through hard work and dedication, he became the Chief of the Fire Prevention Bureau. My mother was a stay-at-home mom. My parents were devout Roman Catholics, and both were active church members. I had one older brother and sister and one younger brother. My parents were loving and caring and were excellent role models. Their hopeful outlook, selflessness, and work ethic inspire me today."

About three weeks after Dr. Byrne was born, FDR's New Deal was implemented to jump-start the economy with help from federal subsidies. To quote the National Archives again:

In his speech accepting the Democratic Party nomination in 1932, Franklin Delano Roosevelt pledged "a New Deal for the American people" if elected. Following his inauguration as President of the United States on March 4, 1933, FDR put his New Deal into action: an active, diverse, and innovative program of economic recovery. In the First Hundred Days of his new administration, FDR pushed through Congress a package of legislation designed to lift the nation out of the Depression. FDR declared a "banking holiday" to end the runs on the banks and created new federal programs administered by so-called "alphabet agencies" …Through employment and price stabilization and by making the government an active partner with the American people, the New Deal jump-started the economy towards recovery.

The New Deal directly impacted Dr. Byrne's father and family. Although it was an entitlement program, the New Deal was structured around the need to work. As second-generation immigrants and devout Roman Catholics, Dr. Byrne's parents were willing to work, and their strength to persevere during the Great Depression was rooted in their Christian faith.

"After I was administered the Sacraments of Baptism, Penance, and first Holy Communion, I served as an altar boy at St. Elizabeth's Church in Norwood," Dr. Byrne recollected. "I received my religious and academic education from the Sisters of Charity at the adjoining grade school with the same name. At twelve, I received the Sacrament of Confirmation at the hands and anointing of Archbishop John McNicholas. Then, in the power of the Holy Spirit, I went to Purcell High School in nearby Cincinnati. Along with learning about my Catholic faith and heritage, my favorite subjects in school were mathematics, science, and English."

"I also enjoyed playing baseball and

basketball, literally basket-ball," Dr. Byrne recalled with a smile. "I cut out the bottom of a bushel basket, climbed a ladder, and nailed it to a telephone pole with a plank for a backboard. I think I spent more time fixing the basket than playing basketball! I was never really good at sports, but they were fun, competitive, and exciting. At the time, we were in the middle of World War II, and the painful realities of the Great Depression were fading away."

Dr. Byrne assisted his father during the war, who taught fire prevention. "I helped my father set up equipment for public address (PA) systems and movies in city parks. We played the *Blondie and Dagwood* comedy movies and followed them with instructions about incendiary bombs. I learned how to speak in public from my father. We also had Victory Gardens. We grew vegetables for canning to feed our family and community and to enable the farmers to provide food for the troops."

Dr. Byrne continued: "I had many jobs growing up. I was a clerk in a deli, worked in a butcher shop, did outdoor work, worked as a car mechanic, and dug graves in a cemetery. All while performing well as a student. I was one of the top thirty students in Cincinnati, so I was chosen to attend a Latin school. I completed six years of schooling in four and graduated high school at sixteen." Soon after, Dr. Byrne went to college, the first child in his family to do so.

He was accepted to Xavier University in Cincinnati for the pre-med program. "My parents encouraged me to become a doctor," he remembered. "Mrs. Cadwallader, an elderly widow of a prominent physician in Norwood, also inspired me. I cut her grass, and after I was done, we would sit and talk about her experiences as a doctor's wife over a glass of ice-cold lemonade. Her husband visited patients in their homes traveling via horse and buggy, and he was often paid with a live chicken! I also had an aunt who was a nun and the administrator of several Mercy Hospitals in and around Cincinnati. We would visit her as a family. These encounters significantly impacted my interest in medicine."

Dr. Byrne shined in the Xavier premed program and received the James T. Cleary Biology Award due to his grasp of the biological sciences. "My thesis was interesting," recalled Dr. Byrne, "because I recorded electrical activity within salamanders intending to develop anticonvulsant medications. Drugs could be studied to maintain normal electrical activity in the altered brain environment, as detected by an electroencephalogram or EEG. This would be crucial in my future calling as a neonatologist and studying brain electrical activity. I developed fine motor skills, gentle hands, and invented micro procedures to work with these tiny creatures."

After being accepted to St. Louis University School of Medicine, Dr. Byrne continued his academic studies, worked hard, and practiced his pro-life Catholic faith. "Between freshman and sophomore year in medical school," Dr. Byrne recalled, "I worked in central supply and an emergency room at a hospital in Cincinnati." He graduated as a Doctor of Medicine (MD) in 1957. Six months later, Dr. Byrne received the Sacrament of Marriage after meeting the love of his life, Shirley.

Dr. Byrne met Shirley during his senior year at medical school. Shirley worked as a nurse in the St. Louis University Hospital orthopedic unit. "Imagine, at the time," Dr. Byrne reflected, "my salary was eighty-five dollars per month; after I was married, my salary jumped to 110 dollars per month! Then, my salary increased incrementally to ten dollars per month annually for the next few years until I became a pediatrician. Shirley worked until our first baby was born, then became a stay-at-home mom."

The couple parented twelve children. "In the first grouping, five of the first six were boys, but the second child to the eldest boy was a girl. Five girls and one boy were in the second grouping," Dr. Byrne smiled. He continued, "What a perfectly ordered family! My daughter Anne Marie, whom you met, is child number nine. Sometimes, it's easier to keep the grouping and number in mind to remember the children, especially now in the later years of life."

"I started the Special Care Nursery at Cardinal Glennon Memorial Hospital for Children about the time of birth of our fifth child," Dr. Byrne recalled. "At that time, I routinely played nine holes of golf every Wednesday with my colleagues. My golfing friends urged me repeatedly to play all eighteen holes with them. One day, I did. I took my clubs home that day and never played golf again! It took too much time away from Shirley and our children; I loved them more than golf."

"I was always an avid fisherman," Dr. Byrne continued. "I thought, 'This would be a great family activity.' I began fishing at fourteen and would do so all day. On his way to work, my father dropped me off at a pay-pond and would pick me up after work. In those days, you paid a dollar to fish and could take four fish home if you caught them. I helped put food on the table by fishing. Also, I learned about a practical and fun activity that several of my children enjoy today."

"As the children grew older," Dr. Byrne went on to say, "since five of the first six children were boys, it was 'natural' to teach them to fish, and eventually, all my children and most of my grandchildren have learned to fish. We had a small Jon Boat where I would take two children to fish at a time. At an agreed-upon one or two hours, I would row back, exchange two children for another set of two, and row back out. As adults, my children love fishing. In the spring, we have an annual family reunion at Bull Shoals Lake in southern Missouri, and we fish to our heart's delight. The fishing event is a family tradition that started sixty years ago. Some of my grandchildren and great-grandchildren join in as well!"

"Of course," Dr. Byrne said, "with all this time around the water fishing, I had to be trained to swim and to teach my children to do so. I learned to swim at thirty when my oldest child was four. I took classes at the YMCA. I've been swimming three miles per week for the past sixty-plus years! Swimming also became a family pastime as well. Since Shirley and I had so many children, the headcount quota was met to open the YMCA pool on Sundays."

"After breakfast and before church on Sundays, I had to round on my sickest patients, which became a family event, too," Dr. Byrne continued. "We packed up the car and headed to the hospital, church, and then to the pool at the YMCA. The hard work and dedication in caring for other people paid off."

Dr. Byrne commented with a beaming complexion: "My oldest son was in the Navy's nuclear power program and spent two years on a submarine. After an honorable discharge, he opened his own computer business. One son is a plumber, another is an artist and real estate broker, and another is in the metal casting business. He really likes to fish," Dr. Byrne said with a chuckle, "so he 'casts' at work and play! My fifth son followed in my footsteps and became a pediatrician. My youngest son is a successful attorney who was recently appointed a judge. Two daughters are special needs educators for disabled children; one has a boutique business, and another is a registered nurse. My other daughters are involved in real estate, childcare, and financial investments."

"The Lord blessed me with twelve wonderful children and a loving and devoted wife," Dr. Byrne commented with gratitude. "Besides my twelve beautiful children, I've also been blessed with thirty-seven grandchildren and seven great-grandchildren. In 2005, my wife, Shirley, received the Sacrament of the Sick and fell asleep in the loving arms of Jesus due to complications from diabetes."

In 1961, Dr. Byrne became an Instructor of Pediatrics at St. Louis University School of Medicine and gradually increased in academic rank to Clinical Professor. In 1963, he received his certification from the American Board of Pediatrics.

"For six years," Dr. Byrne recalled, "I cared for children with leukemia, malignant diseases, and other immune disorders, such as rheumatoid arthritis and lupus. Then, I found my first calling as a physician in 1963 to be a pediatrician specializing in what would eventually become the new subspecialty known as neonatology, which treats prematurely born babies requiring critical care. There was a lot of groundwork before neonatology became an official subspecialty of pediatrics."

Dr. Byrne was appointed Director of the Newborn Nursery at St. Louis University and soon became the Founder and Director of the Neonatal Intensive Care Unit (NICU) at Cardinal Glennon Memorial Hospital for Children. "When I started to specialize in 'neonatology,' the word didn't even exist," Dr. Byrne recollected. "At the time," he continued, "a few doctors in the US and Canada tried to treat prematurely born infants requiring critical care. I was one doctor doing the same thing in St. Louis. Dr. Bob Usher at Toronto Children's Hospital was another, and we became good friends."

Dr. Byrne continued, "Another was Air Force pediatrician Colonel Shepherd, who rounded at my hospital. Work also occurred at Boston Children's Hospital, Vanderbilt University, and Colorado General Hospital. Along with the rise of the subspecialty of neonatology, the evolution of obstetrics, gynecology, and perinatology led to my relationship with Dr. Eugene Hamilton."

Dr. Hamilton was a pioneering obstetrician and medical researcher at St. Mary's Hospital who used serum collected from an Rh-negative mother who had been sensitized by previously carrying an Rh-positive baby. Eventually, this evolved into the development of RhoGAM. This medicine prevents the mother from creating antibodies to attack Rh-positive blood cells in her baby. RhoGAM administered to the mother, initially investigated by Dr. Hamilton, now routinely prevents almost all Rh disease in infants.

The Rhesus factor (Rh) is an antigen found on red blood cells, and it is related to a person's blood type. An incompatible Rh factor between the baby and mother can be severely disabling or deadly to the baby after birth. "The tragic effect," Dr. Byrne said grimly, "the antibodies in the mother destroy the baby's blood cells. The baby then becomes anemic and develops yellow-colored or jaundiced skin due to high bilirubin levels. If not treated with a blood transfusion, the baby can develop debilitating diseases, but most often, they die. RhoGAM prevents this now, but exchange transfusions were first needed to correct the problem *in utero* and *ex utero*."

Dr. Byrne continued: "I worked with Dr. Hamilton during his initial investigations of the Rh factor, and he started with five women who were highly sensitized during a previous pregnancy. During pregnancy, when the baby was identified with Rh disease that could be lethal if not treated, Dr. Hamilton developed a technique to advance a needle through the abdomen of the mother. The procedure to administer the blood transfusion to the baby in the mother's womb was remarkable since this was before ultrasound was used in medical procedures."

Dr. Byrne went on with a note of admiration: "Dr. Hamilton inserted a radio-opaque dye with a needle into the amniotic fluid of the mother's belly. The baby housed in the amniotic sac eventually swallowed the dye with his or her tiny mouth, and the dye was digested and ended up in the baby's abdominal cavity. Using fluoroscopy, a type of x-ray, Dr. Hamilton could now see the dye's location in the baby's belly! This provided the target for inserting the needle to administer the blood transfusion into the baby."

"Dr. Hamilton requested I be present while he delivered these babies," Dr. Byrne continued. "My role was to provide postnatal care and to do the blood exchange transfusion procedure immediately after the birth of the baby. After the umbilical cord was quickly clamped, as was standard practice, I exchanged the Rh-negative blood for the Rh-positive blood. For the transfusion, I inserted a tiny catheter into the umbilical vein of the baby and, with a syringe, removed and infused the blood. Our first two babies died, and we couldn't figure out why. Were the deaths connected to the exchange transfusions?"

"The answer was no," Dr. Byrne continued, "and our knowledge about the deaths came from an unlikely source—lambs. One of the university's animal researchers weighed lambs immediately after birth before the umbilical cord was clamped, and the lambs became heavier during the weighing process. Where did the increased weight come from? Additional blood from blood in the umbilical cord!"

"We also discovered the standard practice of clamping the umbilical cord close to the baby's body did not allow the necessary additional blood from the cord for the newborn baby to provide adequate circulation to sustain their little bodies," Dr. Byrne commented. "The problem was hypovolemia or low blood pressure, circulatory collapse, and respiratory failure that led to death, not complications with the exchange transfusion or Rh-factors. After this problem was ironed out, Dr. Hamilton and I saved the lives of many babies until RhoGAM was created in 1968. For this reason, it is now standard practice to delay clamping of the umbilical cord."

Dr. Byrne exclaimed: "The discovery was terrific, and the opportunity to be involved with Dr. Hamilton's pioneering Rh work was equally fantastic. During that time, I performed many exchange transfusions on babies with Rh disease. Incidentally, my blood is the universal blood type anyone can receive. Multiple times, I went to the lab to donate my blood, then to the nursery to administer my donated blood to babies for life-saving transfusions!"

As a pioneering neonatologist, hard worker, and devout pro-life Roman Catholic, these innovations and medical advances to preserve and protect life were just the beginning for Dr. Byrne, and then he met Joseph.

1

Protector and Defender of Joseph

In 1963, the year President John F. Kennedy was assassinated, Dr. Byrne started the neonatology program at the Cardinal Glennon Memorial Hospital for Children in St. Louis, Missouri. The non-profit institution was founded in 1956 by the Franciscan Sisters of Mary. Cardinal Glennon provides care, often free of charge, to children as it strives to serve in the spirit of the institution's foundress of the Franciscan Sisters, Mother Mary Odilia Berger. In France, the nuns treated smallpox victims and were called the "Smallpox Sisters" as a result. After arriving in St. Louis, this selfless care was transferred to the sick in the

United States (US).

Due to Dr. Byrne's pioneering work and cutting-edge innovation inspired by the Franciscan Sisters, Cardinal Glennon is presently the home of a Level IV neonatal intensive care unit (NICU), the highest designation for infant critical care. Babies requiring a Level IV NICU are born earlier than thirty-two weeks gestation, weigh less than 1,500 grams (roughly the adult human brain's weight), and require ventilator support and other critical care therapies to sustain life.

Aside from his work with Dr. Hamilton, mentioned in the last chapter, Dr. Byrne also established essential lifesaving devices and treatments for preemies. Working with engineers from the NASA space program, he invented a method of recording the blood pressure of these babies. The design of this tiny bicep blood pressure cuff that fits on an astronaut's finger is commonly used on preemies worldwide today. Dr. Byrne also invented a single-unit Infacare incubator monitor that maintained the baby's temperature while monitoring heart rate, respiration, and oxygenation. For these and other revolutionary works in the NICU field, Dr. Byrne was listed with his picture in the "Advances in Medicine" section of the 1973 edition of the *Encyclopedia Americana*.

"When we began," Dr. Byrne recalled, "there were no treatments for preemies and low-birth-weight babies, the type of neonatal care we take for granted today." He continued: "These sick babies had difficulty breathing or other congenital anomalies. Since most died within forty-eight to seventy-two hours, many parents requested Baptism and accepted death. My goal was to do more to honor their God-given life. God called me to be a medical doctor, which meant I had an obligation to treat sick people. What better place to attempt this Holy Spirit-inspired medical ministry than Cardinal Glennon? The institution was already a bastion of God's mercy due to its dedication to the mission of the Sisters of St. Mary."

Dr. Byrne recollected, "As a physician still in training, I vividly remember one of the first pediatric patients I saw. The boy had lead poisoning. His brain had swelled as a result, and he was put on a ventilator to breathe. During those days, the ventilator was a simple cylinder with a piston that forcefully pushed air into the lungs."

Dr. Byrne continued: "I was rounding with

anesthesiologist Dr. John Schweiss, and gazing at the unresponsive boy, I asked him with a note of futility on my breath: 'I said how can this do anything?' Dr. Schweiss responded with a piercing statement that became my mantra as a physician: 'As long as the person is alive, you have to keep trying to figure out what to do until the person dies.'"

"With Dr. Schweiss's words indelibly impressed into my mind as a flashbulb memory," Dr. Byrne soberly stated, "and now, as the director of the newborn nursery at St. Louis University Hospital, I went to the hospital administrator at nearby Cardinal Glennon Memorial Hospital for Children and requested permission to create a center where I could find ways to treat the most vulnerable among us — prematurely born and diseased babies."

The administrator said, "Okay, let's try it for a year."

"During that first year, thirty preemies were referred to me," Dr. Byrne recalled, "and even though most of them died, valuable knowledge about how to treat them was gained."

Dr. Byrne worked with his mentor, Dr.

Schweiss, to create a makeshift breathing apparatus to treat preemies that failed miserably. "This type of 'ventilator,'" Dr. Byrne recalled, "surrounded the baby; it delivered positive pressure into an endotracheal tube to expand the lungs internally and negative pressure outside to try to expand the undeveloped lungs simultaneously. It didn't work."

Dr. Byrne continued: "To measure the pressure gradients, we used a rubber tube from a Bunsen Burner connected to a glass U-tube taped to the nursery wall with a small amount of water that would move with the positive and negative pressure, which would help us measure the pressure in the airway in centimeters of water. It was crazy the stuff we tried to do, but this was before we knew better ways to treat low-birth weight babies requiring critical care."

"Also, in the beginning," Dr. Byrne recalled, "we just put in an umbilical vein catheter and gave doses of bicarbonate to treat unknown levels of acidosis caused by increases in carbon dioxide. In medical school, we learned about the need for acid-base balance in the human body. The ability to measure blood gases occurred in 1958, and shortly after that, blood gas analyzers were developed. However, I could not measure the blood carbon dioxide levels in a preemie's body, which was crucial for treatment."

Dr. Byrne continued, grinning like a Cheshire cat: "I pushed a blood gas machine from the animal laboratory through a tunnel to the nursery, parked it outside, and devised a way to do this with small amounts of blood from the preemies. The nurse on duty scratched her head and wondered: 'What's he up to now?' I believe I was the first physician to perform a blood gas on a preemie in St. Louis. This was an important step in preserving the lives of these babies because now it was possible to analyze the level of carbon dioxide, oxygen, and acidity in their tiny bodies and achieve acid-base balance by administering precise doses of bicarbonate."

Along with the ability to measure acidosis, a critical second step was giving infants positive end-expiratory pressure (PEEP) using constant-flow finely tuned ventilators, which helped "blow off" or reduce acidosis. "Dr. Corcoran, 'Corky,' Rosan was a pathologist at Cardinal Glennon," Dr. Byrne fondly recalled. "Corky was responsible for identifying bronchopulmonary dysplasia or BPD in these newborns, a condition where the baby's undeveloped airways are damaged, and destruction of lung tissue occurs in the alveoli or air sacs where respiration occurs. Too much force from the ventilator can exacerbate this problem by hyper-inflating the lungs, and too little air restricts respiration, results in acidosis, and causes suffocation."

"Thus," Dr. Byrne continued, "I learned a lot about the anatomy and physiology of the lungs and how to treat bronchopulmonary dysplasia and respiratory acidosis using finely tuned respiratory treatments and PEEP. Treating BPD with a ventilator adapted to the lungs of preemies was a game changer. One of the major lessons I learned from Corky was his persistent reminder that a ventilator is not a respirator."

A ventilator moves air into the lungs, and the "respirator" function, or respiration, is a physiological process that occurs in the body — a critical *fundamental* distinction in breathing. The respiratory process in the lungs includes the exchange of oxygen, which is inhaled, and carbon dioxide, which is exhaled. Delivery of air with oxygen is the only thing a ventilator does; respiration and exhalation are functions of the living body. The respiratory and exhalation parts of the body are the same for everyone from birth until death.

Drs. Byrne and Rosan also focused on respiratory distress syndrome in babies treated with too much oxygen. Dr. Byrne explained: "Not only is low oxygen a problem, but too much oxygen can cause problems too. Corky and I collaborated to educate others about respiratory distress syndrome and fine-tuning with the ventilator. Dr. Rosan put together some excellent slides to explain lung function and the pathology of respiratory distress syndrome—I still use many of these images in lectures I give today."

Treating and analyzing preemies effectively required specialized equipment and devices, and this is where the ingenuity, skill, and gentle hands from Dr. Byrne's treatment of salamanders mentioned in the last chapter played a crucial role. Since these babies are so tiny, new, sensitive measurement devices and medical protocols were also needed. We have already considered the NASA-inspired blood pressure cuff and Infacare discoveries. Dr. Byrne and other neonatology pioneers did more, and their dedication to treating these babies improved the practice of medicine worldwide.

Dr. Byrne and colleagues identified the need for magnesium, zinc, and copper in parenteral or intravenous nutrition to meet the metabolic demands of babies. "Our goal was to provide these essential elements intravenously, so we had to create intravenous solutions and tubes that would not irritate or destroy the baby's tiny vein." Microtechniques were developed to measure and quantify magnesium, zinc, and copper from small amounts of urine, stool, and blood (see below). Dr. Byrne and his colleagues developed many other medical treatments beneficial to patients of all ages, not just premies and newborn infants.

"Back then," Dr. Byrne recalled, "seaweed was boiled; the supernatant provided protein to infuse into the infant's vein. We knew seaweed had the necessary protein we wanted. Still, we were oblivious to the concentrations of each batch of seaweed. Eventually, other ways to get protein for intravenous nutrition were developed. Creating total parental nutrition (TPN) with accurate concentrations to meet these babies' metabolic demands was now possible, and these preemies thrived."

Dr. Byrne explained: "For instance, premature infants have minimal total quantities of blood, which required the development of micro techniques to analyze blood for indicators of health or disease." Now, the young and old benefit from these discoveries (e.g., glucometers to test blood glucose), ventilators are more sensitive, and the importance of minerals for the human body are better understood. "It was exciting for me to participate in developing what was then a brand-new field. What you try to accomplish for those sickest people first will ultimately benefit the rest of humanity."

Dr. Byrne concluded: "My medical philosophy is that some of the best doctors are the ones who work the hardest for the sickest people, which was an important lesson I learned from Dr. Schweiss and others at Cardinal Glennon."

After the small beginnings of the neonate unit in 1963 under Dr. Byrne's leadership and modernization, thousands of preemies have been treated at Cardinal Glennon Memorial Hospital for Children. He recalled, "More than 600 babies were referred to me annually from more than fifty hospitals." One patient referred to Dr. Byrne in 1975 was Joseph, and he would define much of Dr. Byrne's subsequent calling as a physician.

Joseph was born very prematurely. "He couldn't breathe or move and was non-responsive to noxious stimuli," Dr. Byrne recollected. "He was on a ventilator," Dr. Byrne continued, "so we did a brainwave test." A brainwave test detects electrical activity in the brain and is called an EEG. "He had a flat electroencephalogram or EEG—in other words, no brainwaves," Dr. Byrne stated. The treating neurologist, the world-renowned Dr. Harvey Sarnat, wrote in Joseph's chart that the finding was "consistent with cerebral death."

Dr. Byrne recalled his exchange with Dr. Sarnat:

"What does this mean, Harvey? I'm not familiar with the diagnosis of cerebral death."

"Oh, don't worry about the finding, Paul. Just wait twenty-four hours and repeat the EEG, and you'll have more information."

"Instead of repeating the EEG in twenty-four hours, as Dr. Sarnat suggested, I performed it after forty-eight hours, and the EEG was unchanged. I asked Dr. Sarnat again for guidance."

"Well, Paul, at some hospitals, they'll turn off the ventilator because the patient does not have detectable activity in the brain. The patient is considered to be in an irreversible coma."

"Harvey, I don't do that. I treat every patient. Some live, some die."

What was evident to Dr. Byrne was that Joseph, whose entire body could be cradled in one hand, still had a beating heart, circulation, and aerating lungs (respiration), even though he was non-responsive and a ventilator supported his breathing. "Joseph had no detectable brain activity, according to Dr. Sarnat, who was no lightweight," Dr. Byrne said solemnly. Yet Joseph was obviously alive.

Dr. Byrne refused to accept Dr. Sarnat's diagnosis and suggestion. He aligned with the desire of Joseph's mother and continued to provide treatment. Not long after, Joseph developed detectable brain activity, arose from his coma, was weaned off the ventilator, and is alive today. "Joseph was on a ventilator for about five weeks and was unresponsive with no detectable brain activity and was not dead, but had an EEG consistent with 'cerebral death.' This would be acceptable to stop his treatment!" Dr. Byrne recalled with a note of irritation in his voice.

"Joseph went on to be a straight-A student in school," an excited Dr. Byrne recalled as he flipped through pictures of him across his lifespan. "He has a successful career," Dr. Byrne continued, "and he's now married and the father of three kids. Removing the ventilator would've ended Joseph's life!" Joseph made Dr. Byrne aware of the unreliability of "brain death" as death. The acceptance of brain death among physicians was disturbing to him.

"In 1975, I didn't know anything about brain death, which was introduced to America seven years prior in 1968. I just continued my practice as a pediatrician specializing in neonatology. I was doing my thing to take care of sick babies and trusted the opinions of my colleagues," Dr. Byrne said.

He continued: "Physicians had a camaraderie

and understanding back then. Each of us did our best to protect and preserve life, so there was a belief that another physician's opinion always favored life and viewed death as a form of defeat. Death imposed on the physician a solemn duty to learn how to prevent it in the future. My belief was Dr. Sarnat shared this conviction."

"Further," Dr. Byrne commented, "when I was in medical school, I was taught it was necessary to wait for the complete absence of all vital bodily functions before declaring death and after that to wait some more. So what were we waiting for? The physician was waiting for the destruction of the brain, heart, and lungs and not just the lack of functions. Joseph lacked detectable neurological activity in his cerebral cortex or the microthin top layer of his brain, only one minuscule part of the vital system, which in time was proved wrong."

"He also had a heart that never stopped and respiration, two chief essential functions for life," Dr. Byrne continued. "Elapsed time also confirmed that Joseph's failure to breathe could be reversed since he developed the ability to inspire. The cart seemed to be moving before the horse in medicine, but maybe Harvey knew something I didn't know about cerebral death as death. I made it my goal to find out if he did."

Dr. Byrne continued: "What I did early on was to look at specific enzymes that are indicators of tissue destruction, particularly creatine phosphokinase, or CPK, an enzyme found primarily in heart, brain, and skeletal muscle. The CPK enzyme that indicates tissue destruction to the brain is called BB, or CK-BB, and it is present after someone has a stroke or other type of brain injury."

"I studied 275 babies," Dr. Byrne reported, "looked at CK-BB, and tried to find a high enough level to indicate total brain destruction. My investigation was futile since no consistent level of the CK-BB emerged to suggest the destruction of brain tissue, much less to serve as a predictor to indicate a progression to the destruction of the brain that would lead to necrosis and death. I tried hard to find a justification for brain death, but my endeavor was unsuccessful. At that point, I realized medicine had changed, and my goal was to dig deeper."

"The significant thing about studies

concerning brain death," Dr. Byrne recalled, "was my desire to investigate it from an academic scientific point of view. I also asked Harvey to direct my reading about brain death since he was a published neurologist, and he referred me to the fund of literature at the time."

According to Anne Hardy and E. M. Tansey, "Medical Enterprise and Global Response: 1945–2000" from *The Western Medical Tradition*, "In the early 1960s, it was agreed that once the brain stem failed, recovery becomes impossible." The authors continue, "With this recognition, the development of specific criteria for brain death developed." In 1966, the French adopted criteria to formulate a clinical definition for brain death or *coma dépussé*, literally translated to English as "a state beyond coma."

A couple of years later, across the Atlantic at Harvard University in Cambridge, Massachusetts, thirteen elites paved the way for a neurological standard to define death in the US. In 1968, the "Report of the Ad Hoc Committee of the Harvard Medical School to Examine the Definition of Brain Death" published its findings in the *Journal* of the *American Medical Association* (*JAMA*) with Dr. Henry Beecher as the lead author. The title of the article was "A Definition of Irreversible Coma."

After researching the subject of death by neurological criteria, including the 1968 Harvard report, Dr. Byrne was shocked by the lack of scientific investigation to establish brain death as *de facto* death. The agreement Anne Hardy and E. M. Tansey wrote about was rooted in other factors, not science. "Brain death was not based on data acceptable for any scientific study," Dr. Byrne commented.

The 1968 Harvard report had no clinical data from patient studies or basic science "experiments on dogs, cats, or rats," Dr. Byrne exclaimed. The report's stated purpose was to redefine death. It aimed to serve the medical community's economic interests, hunger to advance organ transplant research, and to protect doctors who see brain death as death from lawsuits. We'll consider the report from Harvard later in the chapter.

"During my research about brain death," Dr. Byrne recalled, "I noticed that the words functioning, function, destruction, and death were often used interchangeably in the same articles." He explained, "Non-function or functioning refers to idleness or action, not destruction and death. At this point, I soon realized that brain death was rooted in a lot of speculation."

"Three years after Joseph's recovery, I published an article, 'On Death,' in the *Missouri Medicine Journal for the State Medical Society*. Aside from Joseph, part of my inspiration to write this article was influenced by a 1968 episode that indicated prolonged isoelectric or non-detectable EEG data in a patient who fully recovered. The 1968 Harvard committee ignored this remarkable case. Like Joseph, the person had a flat EEG, and he had one for thirty-nine days. Nevertheless, he recovered from the diagnosed 'irreversible coma,' but no one cared," Dr. Byrne exclaimed.

Dr. Byrne continued: "There were also a couple of studies after 1968 before the redefinition of death in 1981 that did not support brain death as death. These findings were also ignored. In 1971, the EEGs of nine patients diagnosed brain dead were looked at, and two of the nine still had EEG activity." Roughly 20 percent still had detectable electrical activity—this should have raised an eyebrow. Perhaps the rest of those studied would have developed electrical activity over time, or maybe the conviction that the EEG equipment was not sensitive enough to detect brainwaves in the seven others (two plausible assumptions). However, the conclusion, "It was no longer required to do brainwave testing to determine brain death," Dr. Byrne said with notable irritation.

In late 1970, the *New England Journal of Medicine* (*NEJM*) published a two-part article, "Brain Death," by Dr. Peter Black. Ten years had elapsed since Dr. Beecher's Harvard report, and thirty disparate sets of brain-death criteria were used in the US. When medical science is applied, a best practice develops, and the thirty dissimilar sets of unique brain-death criteria underscore the lack of empirical consensus among physicians. Dr. Byrne recalled, "I was inspired to write an extensive article as a two-part series in a similar way, but the *NEJM* refused to publish it. At about the same time, the neurologist Dr. Earl Walker published the first edition of his highly influential *Cerebral Death*."

The most extensive study was conducted in

1977 by the National Institutes of Health (NIH). This study was called the "Collaborative Study," and "it was published piece-mail in multiple journals," Dr. Byrne recalled. "I had to go from journal to journal to find the results." The study reported on "503 patients" that met brain-death criteria, and "forty-four didn't die, and those 226 who did die, they looked at the brain, and 10 percent had no gross pathology in the brain, yet they were declared brain dead." As for the remaining 233, they died, but no autopsy was performed.

Dr. Byrne realized then "that brain death is a mendacity or falsehood, a deception, a lie, and it was made up. I contacted the NIH to request the 'Collaborative Study' be published in one place so that others could be aware of the lack of science behind using brain death to define death. As a government institution serving the public, the NIH was required to publish 100 copies of the study, but they refused to publish more than that amount."

Other factors were in play, and foremost was the desire to harvest healthy organs to transplant, as the 1968 Harvard report laid out as "primary purpose" number two: "Obsolete criteria for the definition of death can lead to controversy in obtaining organs for transplantation."

Dr. Christiaan Barnard performed the first human-to-human heart transplant at the Groote Schuur Hospital in Cape Town, South Africa. On December 3, 1967, Dr. Barnard cut the heart out of a twenty-five-year-old woman, Denise Darvall, who was hit by a car and suffered a head injury, and transplanted it into Lewis Washkansky, a fifty-four-year-old South African grocer with heart disease and diabetes.

Dr. Barnard told Washkansky that the transplant surgery had an 80 percent chance of success, which it did not. Also, rather than wait for Darvall's heart to stop beating, he caused a cardiac arrest using potassium, declared her dead, and restarted her heart. At the time, removing vital organs from people with a beating heart was illegal. Washkansky lived only eighteen days after the heart transplant, but Dr. Barnard was not deterred. Instead, he pursued his medical malpractice with greater vigor.

On January 2, 1968, Dr. Barnard attempted a second heart transplant. The recipient was a retired white dentist, Philip Blaiberg, who survived for nineteen months. The donor was a twenty-four-year-old black man, Clive Haupt, who suffered a brain bleed while picnicking with his family. Haupt's attending physician, Dr. Bill Hoffenberg, was approached by Dr. Barnard's transplant team, and they asked him to declare Haupt dead. Hoffenberg recoiled at the request to proclaim a breathing and heart-beating man dead but eventually recanted.

Dr. Barnard's eagerness to succeed in human-to-human heart transplants was not homegrown. He studied medicine at the University of Cape Town but received his heart transplant training in the US. In 1955, Dr. Barnard relocated to Minnesota to further his studies at the State's university, where he was introduced to the heart-lung machine or cardiopulmonary bypass pump invented by Dr. John Gibbon in 1953.

The machine's function is to keep the person's body perfused with oxygen-rich blood during cardiac surgery while the heart is stopped. Soon after, Dr. Barnard studied and practiced medicine under the guidance of Dr. Walt Lillehei, an open-heart surgery pioneer. Upon returning to South

Africa in 1958, Barnard was appointed head of the Department of Experimental Surgery at the Groote Schuur Hospital, Cape Town.

Heart transplant surgery research started in the US during the 1950s. American surgeon Dr. Norman Shumway, also trained under Dr. Lillehei, performed a dog-to-dog heart transplant at Stanford University in California in 1958. The first successful human transplant surgery in America was a kidney transplant performed by Dr. Joseph Murray in 1954, in which both donor and recipient, who were identical twins, continued to live for several years.

The transplant race was on, and morals and ethics were lowered as the hunger for organs increased. In 1966, the same year Drs. Shumway and Barnard met again at Standford University, Drs. Lillehei and William Kelly transplanted a pancreas. Dr. Barnard returned to South Africa in 1967 and performed the heart transplant mentioned above. However, three days after Bernard's operation, a gruesome and evil heart transplant surgery occurred at Maimonides Medical Center in Brooklyn, New York.

Dr. Adrian Kantrowitcz performed the second

heart transplant surgery on December 6, 1967, just three days after Dr. Barnard's first heart transplant. Dr. Byrne shared a picture of a three-day-old baby in a stainless-steel pan packed with ice. The baby looked like every other sleeping infant with closed eyes but had a tube in his mouth. His body was submerged in ice cubes that looked like large blocks compared to his tiny frame. The still-living baby performed respiration, circulation, and exhalation until butchered to death by Dr. Kantrowitcz.

A disturbed Dr. Byrne stated with disgust and anger: "They cut the beating heart out of a three-day-old baby and transplanted it into an eighteen-day-old baby. They decided they could take the heart of the three-day-old baby because he was mentally impaired, and the eighteen-day-old baby was more entitled to it because he was not mentally disabled. At the end of those capers, both babies were dead. It was illegal and immoral, so they had to do something. So, what did they do? They set up a committee, the Harvard committee, and invented brain death!"

As noted above, Dr. Beecher led the charge as the committee chairman. He was a respected professor of anesthesiology at Harvard University Medical School at the time and a leading physician in the US. The Upjohn Company organized a conference on March 22, 1964, and invited him to speak. An eager Dr. Beecher accepted the invitation and alerted the conference organizers that he had a self-designated "bombshell" speech to deliver.

Indeed, Dr. Beecher's bold talk blasted his colleagues for unethical research, but he conveniently omitted his egregious human rights abuses. During this speech, he commented on the abrogation of responsibility among American researchers for not providing informed consent to research subjects. He cited twenty-two examples in the published medical literature but conveniently omitted his own immoral, unethical, and uninformed research he performed on human beings.

In post-war Germany, Dr. Beecher conducted human experiments with drugs in collaboration with the Central Intelligence Agency (CIA). These experiments and interrogations, which could be described as torture, occurred at a covert CIA interrogation site in Kronberg, Germany, on the outskirts of Frankfurt. According to witnesses, Dr. Beecher's drug experiments resulted in the deaths of several interrogated. Also, he met with the Nazi Dr. Walter Schreiber for an "exchange of ideas," which Dr. Schreiber described as "intelligent and cooperative."

After returning to the United States, Dr. Beecher continued his experimental research with drugs, this time LSD (lysergic acid diethylamide, a mind-altering drug that may cause severe paranoia). A 1956 article published in the *Journal of Clinical and Experimental Psychopathology* examined the effects of LSD on different personality types, and he used his students as guinea pigs. According to Dr. Beecher, one of the research subjects exhibited a "vasomotor disturbance with pallor, cold, clammy skin, nonpalpable pulse, slight convulsive movement of the face, and stiffening of the body."

Yet, he continued his human research without providing informed consent. Dr. Beecher did not mention these glaring human rights violations in his speech. He was about to embark on another hypocrisy that would redefine death with inspiration from Nazi Germany rooted in a policy called *Lebensunwertes Leben,* a phrase translated into English as "life unworthy of life."

Drs. Schreiber and Beecher were acquainted with this idea. This 1920 doctrine permitted euthanasia for people with congenital abnormalities, developmental problems, and mental impairment. The ideas undergirding the *Lebensunwertes Leben* gave rise to the horrors of Nazism and an attempt to exterminate the Jews. Approximately six million Jews, 5,000 children born with genetic deficits, and 200,000 people with neurocognitive problems met their demise under *Lebensunwertes Leben* policies. The program was directed and supervised by medical doctors in Germany, including Dr. Schrieber, a brigadier-general of the Wehrmacht Medical Service.

Some of the *Lebensunwertes Leben* ideas were also supported in America in the early twentieth century. In 1916, eugenics supporter and founder of Planned Parenthood, Margaret Sanger, established the nation's first "birth control clinic" to cleanse the American gene pool. In a 1957 interview with Mike Wallace, she stated: "I believe the greatest sin in the world is bringing children into the world—that have diseases from their parents, that have no chance in the world to be a human being practically."

According to Sanger, the US government must eliminate these children born to "feebleminded" or "imbecilic" parents. Her agenda was triumphant. In 1927, the United States Supreme Court ruled to permit compulsory sterilization for people deemed "unfit," and roughly 70,000 "imbeciles" were sterilized. Then, in 1973, the Supreme Court ruled to allow on-demand abortion—Sanger's lethal assault on unborn life. Before laws to protect the evil of abortion, however, the other attack was Dr. Beecher's "A Definition of Irreversible Coma" in 1968.

The document undergirding the *Lebensunwertes Leben* policy was *The Permission to Destroy Life Unworthy of Living*, and the similarities it shares with the "Report of the Ad Hoc Committee of the Harvard Medical School to Examine the Definition of Brain Death" are shocking. Reputable experts in their respective fields wrote both documents. These elites discuss physicians' legal role in determining the line between life and death, the futility of care for those in altered mental states, the economic burden these people cause to society, and how others deemed more worthy to live on can benefit from them.

The Permission to Destroy Life Unworthy of Living, comments Robert Jay Lifton in his 1986 *New York Times Magazine* article, "German Doctors and the Final Solution," revealed that "a policy of killing was compassionate and consistent with medical ethics." He says the authors "pointed to situations where doctors were obliged to destroy life—interrupting a pregnancy to save the mother, for example."

Further, the writers of the paper "claim that various forms of psychiatric disturbance, brain damage, and retardation indicated that the patients were already 'mentally dead,'" notes Lifton. The authors of the manifesto "characterized these people as 'human ballast' and 'empty shells of human beings.'" According to the writers, Lifton continued, ending these people's lives "is not to be equated with other types of killing [and it is] an allowable, useful act."

"A Definition of Irreversible Coma: Report of the Ad Hoc Committee of the Harvard Medical School to Examine the Definition of Brain Death" states:

> Our primary purpose is to define irreversible coma as a new criterion for death. There are two reasons why there is a need for a definition: (1) Improvements in resuscitative and supportive measures have led to increased efforts to save those who are desperately injured. Sometimes these efforts have only partial success so that the result is an individual whose heart continues to beat but whose brain is irreversibly damaged. The burden is great on patients who suffer permanent loss of intellect, on their families, on the hospitals, and on those in need of hospital beds already occupied by these comatose patients. (2) Obsolete criteria for the definition of death can lead to controversy in obtaining organs for transplantation.

The Committee desires to redefine death for those in a "coma" that a *physician decides* is "irreversible," or to put it in the words of the Nazis, in a "mentally dead" state. These unresponsive people are nothing more than heart-beating corpses dependent on a ventilator. Dr. Beecher agrees with the Nazi physicians; they're just "human ballasts" and "empty shells of human beings." They are a burden "on their families, on the hospitals, and those in need of hospital beds" due to their "loss of intellect," and, therefore, ending their lives is "an allowable, useful act."

Nevertheless, those *a physician judges* as "mentally dead" are valuable to society since they possess perfused organs that can be transplanted into those deemed more worthy to live. If an "irreversible coma [is] a new criterion for death," we can legally murder these people by cutting out their healthy hearts, lungs, livers, kidneys, and other organs. Harvesting organs from these people "is not to be equated with other types of killing." Dr. Beecher was blunt and candid in a 1967 lecture: "Can society afford to discard the tissues and organs of the hopelessly unconscious patient when they could be used to restore the otherwise hopelessly ill but salvageable individual?"

As for more specifics, the Harvard report commented on the historical understanding of death and legal issues associated with the definition of death to make its case to redefine death, but the assertions are specious.

From ancient times down to the recent past it was clear that, when the respiration and heart stopped, the brain would die in a few minutes; so the obvious criterion of no heart beat as synonymous with death was sufficiently accurate. In those times the heart was considered to be the central organ of the body; it is not surprising that its failure marked the onset of death.

While the absence of breathing and a beating heart were indicators of death in "ancient times," no one back then believed "the brain would die in a few minutes." *The brain did not enter the picture until the mechanistic anthropology of the eighteenth century and the rise of materialism in the nineteenth.*

Concerning the "heart" as the "central organ of the body," the ancients did not have in mind the cardiac muscle pumping oxygenated blood throughout the body; instead, they thought about the spirit or soul as an *immaterial life force* that *gave life to the body as a whole unit*. The Harvard committee rewrote thousands of years of history. The group made it look like the ancients accepted a view of death where the brain was involved, which was simply not the case.

The "Legal Commentary" section mentions two cases the courts had to rule on to decide if death occurred. In both cases, there was a need to appeal to physicians for expert testimony. According to the 1951 edition of *Black's Law Dictionary*, which the Committee cited, the standard legal definition for death was defined as: "The cessation of life; the ceasing to exist; *defined by physicians* as a total stoppage of the circulation of the blood, and a cessation of the animal and vital functions consequent thereupon, such as respiration, pulsation, etc [italics added]." The Harvard committee added the italics to emphasize that the physician determines death.

Since "it was agreed" among physicians, as Hardy and Tansey assumed earlier in the chapter, that "brain death" equaled death, *Black's* definition of death was insufficient because expert testimony could conflict with the law of the land.

At present, the law of the United States, in all 50 states and in the federal courts, treats the question of human death as a question of fact to be decided in every case. When any doubt exists, the courts seek medical expert testimony concerning the time of death of the particular individual involved. However, the law makes the assumption that the medical criteria for determining death are settled, and not in doubt among physicians.

As the "patient's condition can be determined only by a physician," argues the committee, consistent guidelines are needed for physicians affirming brain death as death. They should be afforded legal protection for declaring living people dead and not charged with murder for cutting out their vital living organs, which is the crux of the whole matter.

The Harvard Committee succeeded in its purpose of redefining death to protect brain-death-dealing doctors thirteen years later, but not before Dr. Byrne and colleagues published "Brain Death—An Opposing Viewpoint" in a 1979 edition of *JAMA*, the subject of the next chapter.

2

"Brain Death — An Opposing Viewpoint"

One of the problems with organ transplants is that the recipient's body rejects them. "The same is true when a woman gets pregnant," Dr. Byrne commented, "but God created a way for the mother's immune system to be turned down so she can carry her baby. The same is not true when someone receives an organ from another person."

In 1979, all of this would change with the discovery of cyclosporin, a Norwegian fungus. Cyclosporin, now the name for the generic medication, has an immunosuppressant effect on the recipient's body, preventing organ rejection.

Nothing stopped organ transplant surgeries now, but another significant problem needed to be addressed — the requirement of perfused organs — which meant redefining death and a statute to permit anatomical gifts.

As noted in the last chapter, Dr. Beecher led the charge with "A Definition of Irreversible Coma" in 1968. Two years later, Kansas became the first state to pass a statute to permit a definition of death as brain death. In 1975, the Law and Medicine Committee of the American Bar Association (ABA) drafted a Model of Definition of Death Act to include a neurological standard to define death. In 1978, the National Conference of Commissioners on Uniform State Laws (NCCUSL) or Uniform Law Commission (ULC) drafted the Uniform Brain Death Act.

Then, in 1979, the American Medical Association (AMA) created its Model Determination of Death statute based on neurological criteria. In the meantime, twenty-five state legislatures adopted laws based on these existing brain-death models. The redefinition of death became a model law at the 1980 meeting of the NCCUSL or ULC in Kaui, Hawaii, as the 1981 Uniform

Determination of Death Act (UDDA).

During this time, Dr. Byrne's medical career was flourishing. He was a respected pediatrician specializing in neonatology and was published in peer-reviewed journals. Dr. Byrne's advocacy for the lives of those in vulnerable conditions shifted into high gear in the 1970s. As a result of his diligent pro-life activity, he was elected vice president of the medical staff at Cardinal Glennon Memorial Hospital for Children. He served simultaneously as the Director of St. Louis University Perinatal Center for Southern Illinois, a position he would hold until 1980.

Dr. Byrne received his neonatal and perinatal medicine certification from the American Academy of Pediatrics (AAP) in 1975 — the first official board exam and certification offered for that pediatric subspecialty. Six in St. Louis took the exam, and Dr. Byrne was one of two who passed. In 1978, the AMA called on him to participate in a panel discussion about "Ethical Issues in the Care of the Small Premature."

While Dr. Byrne's career as a neonatologist was essential to him, the Holy Spirit kept nudging him to confront the growing acceptance of brain death. How could he not be bothered after watching Joseph fully recover and experiencing his electroencephalogram (EEG) report as "consistent with cerebral death"? The neurologist judged Joseph to be in Dr. Beecher's "irreversible coma" and, therefore, "mentally dead" and not worthy of ongoing care and treatment.

In 1979, Dr. Byrne published "Brain Death—An Opposing Viewpoint" with two colleagues in the *Journal of the American Medical Association* (*JAMA*). Dr. Byrne wrote the article with Dr. Sean O'Reilly, Department of Neurology, George Washington Medical Center, and Paul M. Quay, S.J., Ph.D., Department of Theological Studies and Physics, St. Louis University. The article was written to stop the move to redefine death with neurological criteria, and it does so by pointing out several fallacies that undergird using brain-related criteria to determine whether death has occurred.

The authors write:

In a 1977 article in the [*JAMA*], Veith [and colleagues] argued in support of defining death by statute. They favored, in particular, a statute modeled on the American Bar Association's (ABA's) proposed definition of death: "For all legal purposes, a human body with irreversible cessation of total brain function, according to usual and customary standards of medical practice, shall be considered dead. ...The present article is written to show that the ABA's definition of death and, indeed, all 19 or so statutes that have undertaken to define and establish at law "brain-related" criteria of death are based on scientifically invalid assumptions and are also opposed to the three major religious traditions of this country.

A significant part of the article points out the "scientifically invalid assumptions" that equate brain death with death, and it briefly addresses, but no less cogently, how a neurological definition of death opposes traditional religious beliefs.

The first line of defense for life begins with defining death as an observed state of being. Then, the article shows how supporters of brain death conflate "context-dependent definitions" of death and equate them with science when they are *a priori* assumptions.

When speaking of "definitions of death," a sharp distinction must be made between two quite different modes of definition. On the one hand, "death" is the word we use *to name* a certain *empirically given* state of affairs, a state difficult to describe in full generality, yet one with which we are all too familiar as a situation of fact. Someone we have known ceases to breathe, sags wherever not supported; we find no pulse; there is no sign of inner activity or of reaction; all is silent, inert, then cold; the body grows rigid, later becomes flaccid and begins to putrefy, decomposing till only bones remain. Most importantly, from a certain moment on—"the moment of death"—whatever happens …is entirely describable in terms of disintegration, dissolution, destruction of the unity of the single organism that was formerly present: a human being has, so far as this world can tell, simply ceased to be.

Actual death is an observable state. A line is crossed from life to death, and this new mode of being can be scientifically proven. Death can also be redefined, but this redefinition of death will be driven by a worldview rooted in *a priori* assumptions, not *a posteriori* experience—empirical fact. "The shallow approach to so profound a reality as death taken by a number of medical and legal ethicists today who consider death not to be a fact but a matter of mere use of convenient language or convenient social stipulations seems to arise from their confounding the two basic kinds of definitions," the authors noted.

Now, at law, the nonempirical, context-related definitions of philosophers and theologians have in the past been carefully avoided, if for no other reason than that it is not within the competence of the law to discriminate among them. But death itself, the fact, not the concept, the endlessly repeated and sorrow-laden seeming extinction of human beings, *is* the law's concern as it is that of the ordinary people who look to the law for the protection of their lives. No moving away from the *empirical* notion of death can be acceptable at law.

The authors then carefully point out: "The legal question being debated at present ...is not about the definition of death, despite the efforts of some to turn it that way, but about the validity of certain proposed *generalized criteria* for death."

At this point, the second argument for defending life is set into motion. "Now," the authors contend, "most of the 'definitions of death' under current discussion, eg, irreversible cessation of total brain function, turn out to be, on inspection, just such general criteria."

All general criteria used as standard up to now have developed from the intention to make sure that a person who is still alive will not be treated as if dead. The proposed new criteria are intended to be used in the opposite sense: to prevent someone from being treated as alive when he is already dead. One is concerned now to prevent the possibility that present day life-support systems might mask death and cause a corpse to mimic life—at the expense to the living, in suffering and money. In the past, a mistaken determination of death usually had no other result for a dying patient than his being allowed to die without further treatment. But the new criteria are intended not only to decide as soon as possible when someone is dead but, among other options, to clear the way for the excision of his vital organs—action which, if a mistake has been made, is certain to kill the still living patient. …the proposed criteria are far less certain than the older ones; they are, we shall argue, not merely uncertain but certainly wrong in principle.

"We point out first that nothing describable as 'brain function' is simply equivalent to human life," the authors continue. Further, the authors "argue that cessation of function, whether irreversible or not, has no necessary connection with either destruction of the brain or death of the person and, therefore, cannot serve as a general criterion of death."

The brain consists not of a single part but of several closely interrelated ones (cortex, cerebellum, midbrain, medulla, etc). Though composed of superficially similar tissues and closely linked together both anatomically and physiologically, yet these parts can continue to live and act independently of one another, even when one or more of them has been destroyed. As one might then expect, the brain as a whole has no physiologically identifiable, single function that could be called the "life-giving function" or the function of the brain as "organ of the whole." Rather, there exists a large multiplicity of different functions that are characteristic of the different parts. Although the characteristic functions of the brain-parts normally are closely coordinated, each part can function without the others. Further, none of these parts is in complete control of the others.

Thus, arguing that death equals the loss of brain function is a *non-sequitur* since no single brain process can be defined as a life-giving function for human beings.

The brain is, then, an organ whose varied functions serve to integrate physiologically (eg, by biophysical, biochemical, or other neuronal mechanisms) the different parts of the body. Such physiological operations of integration are, in fact, the ordinary conditions for the continuance of the organismic unity of the body. But if "total brain function" can legitimately mean no more than the sum total of the characteristic functions of all parts of the brain, then the brain's ceasing to function does not imply, a priori, its destruction but only its loss of physiological activity.

The authors admit that death will follow if the *destruction* of the brain occurs by this physiological disruption of function. It is "the total destruction of the entire brain" that validates the "irreversible cessation of every kind of brain function." People with loss of brain function may be dying. Still, it is uncertain if their condition is irreversible and if the *destruction* of their entire brain will occur. "Therefore," the authors continue, "there is no reason to think that cessation of function, whether reversible or irreversible, necessarily implies total or even partial destruction of the brain; still less, death of the person."

Thus, the statutes that have sought to turn a loss of brain function into a general criterion of death are all vitiated by a fundamental category mistake: they take *that which functions* to be simply identical with its *functioning*. Yet, if something irreversibly ceases to function, its existence is not necessarily extinguished, thereby; it merely becomes permanently idle. Non-function, no matter what qualifiers are used with it, is not the same thing as destruction.

"In such circumstances," the authors insist, "one would certainly not be free to treat a patient as dead." If the patient loses function, then "we are dealing with a living patient" with a loss of the capacity to function at that moment in time, and "by this very fact he is not yet dead," but in a state of idleness.

The third line of defense for life is the noun qualifier "irreversibility," which is a scientifically bankrupt term—a presumption—and "insufficient ground for removing a patient's vital organs or the immediate autopsy, cremation, or burial."

Now, irreversibility as such is not an empirical concept and cannot be empirically determined. Both destruction of the brain and the cessation of its function are, in principle, directly observable; such observations can serve as evidence. Irreversibility, however, of any kind, is a property about which we can learn only by inference from prior experience. It is not an observable condition. Hence, it cannot serve as evidence, nor can it rightly be made part of an empirical criterion of death.

"In brief," the authors summarize, "to regard irreversibility of cessation of brain function (at best, a deduction from a set of symptoms) as synonymous or interchangeable with the destruction of the entire brain (one but not the only possible cause of these symptoms) is to commit a compound fallacy: identifying the symptoms with their cause when several are possible." The *etiology* for the "irreversible" symptoms is not known; therefore, *no diagnosis* can be made.

The fourth and final line of defense for life is aimed at those who profess belief in the existence of a soul, spirit, or immaterial life force distinct from the brain.

Philosophically, the [brain death] argument implies, all unnoticed by many of its proponents, a strict materialism. It reduces life of the human person to a putative organic function of the material brain. "Brain function" is so defined as to take the place of the immaterial principle or "soul" of man. Of course, such materialism is a widely held philosophical option. But it stands in flat contradiction to the religious beliefs of Christians, Jews, Moslems, Hindus, and many others. Thus, no arguments based on such reasoning can be allowed if religious acceptability is claimed, as it has been by Veith [and colleagues].

Veith and his colleagues undermine their position when they argue: "Thus, *destruction of the entire brain, and only that*, is consonant with biblical pronouncements on what constitutes an acceptable definition of death," the authors quote him as saying with emphasis added. Veith and colleagues then go on to *conflate the destruction of the brain with the loss of brain function*, which brings us back to the second argument mentioned above.

The central religious beliefs in the United States (US) affirm the existence of things outside the physical world, like God, angels, souls, spirits, or a life force, and philosophical materialism patently rejects the metaphysical or supernatural.

As many others before them have done, Veith [and colleagues] discuss medical feasibility and write at length concerning legal advantages. What seems to be novel in their article are their arguments that "pronouncements of death on brain-related criteria are in accord with secular philosophy and principles of the three major Western religions."

Veith and colleagues made a superficial study of the three major Western religions, especially since each one—Islam, Judaism, and Christianity—has traditionally affirmed divine revelation and the existence of the supernatural. What is surprising is how many lawyers, doctors, and ethicists who profess a belief in one of the three major religions have accepted brain death as death. "Here," the authors conclude, "suffice it to remark that we would do better to work at repeal of current legislation on the subject rather than extend it further."

Even after pointing out how scientifically, logically, and religiously unsound brain death as a definition of death was, their article fell on deaf ears. As noted above, in 1980, the NCCUSL convened and drafted the Uniform Determination of

Death Act (UDDA) in Kauai, Hawaii. The Act received approval from the AMA and the ABA, and the model statute was adopted in 1981 as federal law.

All fifty states affirmed the UDDA with minor variations. The Act is as follows:

An individual who has sustained either (1) irreversible cessation of circulatory and respiratory functions, or (2) irreversible cessation of all functions of the entire brain, including the brain stem, is dead. A determination of death must be made in accordance with accepted medical standards.

Dr. Beecher's horrible life-denigrating dream was codified as US law. Dr. Byrne, however, would not give up the fight to protect and preserve life. He received the prestigious Cardinal Carberry Award in 1979 for his dogged pro-life activity against the growing culture of death in the US.

"I'm a patriotic person," Dr. Byrne commented, "I believe all men are created equal and endowed with certain unalienable rights: life, liberty, and the pursuit of happiness." In traditional medicine, "the rights of a patient are based on human nature and natural moral law," Dr. Byrne said.

"Natural law is about how God is inside each of us. He is inside every human being, and natural moral law has to do with how we deal with each person because of this reality."

Dr. Byrne recited the Preface to the United States Constitution again and said: "Unalienable rights mean they're there, they're right with us. When God creates us, not only does he create the soul, intellect, and will, but he also gives those rights to each person in the womb. The individual's right to life is fundamental because everything our Constitution grants hinges on this God-given right," Dr. Byrne concluded.

The UDDA does not respect a person's right to life and violates the Constitution. In July of 1981, the President's Commission for the Study of Ethical Problems in Medicine and Biomedical and Behavioral Research drafted *Defining Death: Medical, Legal and Ethical Issues in the Determination of Death* and approved the UDDA. The Preface underscores the concerns raised by Dr. Byrne in his 1979 *JAMA* article.

The interest in these statutes arises from modern advances in lifesaving technology. A person may be artificially supported for respiration and circulation after all brain functions cease irreversibly. The medical profession, also, has developed techniques for determining loss of brain functions while cardiorespiratory support is administered. At the same time, the common law definition of death cannot assure recognition of these techniques. The common law standard for determining death is the cessation of all vital functions, traditionally demonstrated by "an absence of spontaneous respiratory and cardiac functions." There is, then, a potential disparity between current accepted biomedical practice and the common law.

As Dr. Byrne and his colleagues noted, there is no way to know if all brain functions have irreversibly ceased in a person with a beating heart, circulation, and aerating lungs (respiration) on a ventilator. Medical technology, ventilators, and drugs do not mask death and require a still-living person to work! Further, no new "developed techniques exist for determining loss of brain functions while cardiorespiratory support is administered" other than those that can objectively measure the destruction of the entire brain, not the loss of its functions.

The Presidential Commission was biased and insisted on endorsing the Beecher doctrine and concocting a "socially-accepted basis for making determinations of death" that reflects the tactics, aims, and goals used in Nazi Germany. One that violates American citizens' unalienable right to "life," which the US Constitution is supposed to protect, along with "liberty and the pursuit of happiness."

Eight years after Roe vs. Wade, death was now redefined with a neurological standard, and people could be put to death by removing their vital organs and giving them to those judged more worthy to live. Medical institutions would rake in billions of dollars on the backs of these *uninformed* organ donors, who were manipulated by deceptive organ procurement propaganda and the capitalist goals of the NCCUSL, AMA, ABA, and Ronald Reagan's 1981 Commission.

Dr. Byrne upheld the Constitution and fought with all his might to defend life. War was waged against life with the legalization of abortion in 1973 and now the legal fiction of the UDDA in 1981.

After relocating to Nebraska, Dr. Byrne continued his career as a pro-life physician and member of the state's American Academy of Pediatrics (AAP) from 1981 to 1986. He served as a clinical professor of pediatrics at Creighton University School of Medicine and as the director of neonatology at Archbishop Bergan Mercy Hospital during those same years. Soon after, Dr. Byrne joined the Fellowship of Catholic Scholars. Then, in 1982, he wrote a letter to the editor of *JAMA* to confront the slippery slope of "The Uniform Anatomical Gift Act" (UAGA).

The UAGA was set into motion in 1967 by the NCCUSL, one year before Dr. Beecher's "A Definition of Irreversible Coma," for the sole purpose of the exploitative bloody harvest. The Act provides a regulatory framework for donating organs, tissues, and other human body parts in the US. The UAGA was adopted by every state, including the District of Columbia, within three years after the NCCUSL or ULC approved it. Dr. Byrne was writing to the *JAMA* Council on Scientific Affairs by addressing the issue of organ donor recruitment, presumed consent, and the chain of people who may donate other people's body parts.

He writes:

Reference is made to the Uniform Anatomical Gift Act (UAGA), which does not always involve "donation." The UAGA takes away the individual's right to refuse being an organ donor unless there is available an "actual notice of contrary indications by the decedent." In the absence of such actual notice, there is incorporated into the UAGA a descending order of classes of persons who may grant authority for use of "all or any part of the decedent's body," eventually reaching "any other person authorized or under obligation to dispose of the body." Furthermore, "the persons authorized ...may make the gift after death or immediately before death." While the UAGA does not distinguish these two states, there is certainly a difference from the point of view of the defenseless individual.

While a superficial read of the UAGA appears to support an "opt-in" system for organ donation, subtle language also erodes the right to life for the "defenseless individual," whether in the womb or on a ventilator. Dr. Byrne points this out by quoting sections of the model form of the 1968 UAGA. The UAGA would be revised in 1987 and again in 2006. Dr. Byrne had the foresight in 1982 to see the ongoing erosion of people's unalienable rights.

The 2006 NCCUSL or ULC states the following:

The two previous anatomical gift acts, as well as this [Act], adhere to an "opt in" principle as its default rule. Thus, an individual becomes a donor only if the donor or *someone acting on the donor's behalf affirmatively makes an anatomical gift*. The system universally adopted in this country is contrary to the system adopted in some countries, primarily in Europe, where an individual is deemed to be a donor unless the individual or another person acting on the individual's behalf "opts out." This other system is known as "presumed consent." While there are proponents of presumed consent who believe the concept of presumed consent could receive in the future a favorable reception in this country, the professional consensus appears to be not to replace the present opt-in principle at this time (emphasis mine).

"This is simply not the case," comments Dr. Byrne. Again, the language is subtle in this sixty-four-page revision. Definitions are important.

On page sixteen of the document, it states the following:

"Prospective donor" means an individual who is dead *or near death and has been determined by a procurement organization to have a part* that could be medically suitable for transplantation, therapy, research, or education. The term does not include an individual who has made a refusal. ..."*Refusal*" *means a record created* under Section 7 *that expressly states an intent to bar other persons from making an anatomical gift of an individual's body or part* (emphasis mine).

Dr. Byrne explains: "Your refusal for organ donation must be documented," as noted above. He continued: "According to the revised Anatomical Gift Act language, you must document your refusal, or opt-out, in writing using explicit language; otherwise, it is presumed that you have consented to be an organ donor to be utilized for organ transplantation, therapy, research, or education."

In addition, organ procurement organizations may identify prospective donors in hospital beds, approach traumatized and bewildered family members, and pressure them to give the gift of the vulnerable loved one's life. These procurement specialists are experts trained in techniques to make a seemingly futile situation seem more meaningful by donating organs. They prey on the altruism of uninformed registered organ donors and traumatized family members.

The organs and tissues from one organ donor will rake in billions for transplant centers and physicians, so exploitation is a genuine concern. "In the absence of such actual notice," Dr. Byrne wrote as we zoom in on his primary concern, "there is incorporated into the UAGA a descending order of classes of persons who may grant authority for use of 'all or any part of the decedent's body,' eventually reaching 'any other person authorized or under obligation to dispose of the body'" even a hospital administrator, who definitely has a conflict of interest. The UAGA is a convoluted and confusing social contract that exploits uninformed, vulnerable people — the devil is in the details.

Dr. Byrne's defense for life pivoted to defending the unalienable rights of defenseless organ donors by confronting the UAGA. However, the fiercest fighting was still against the frontline assault on life by the UDDA. One surprising twist in redefining death was the acceptance of brain-death criteria by some in the visible Body of Christ, the Holy Catholic Church.

All Christians affirm fundamental truths about life, death, and the resurrection of the body, whether Roman Catholic, Protestant, or Orthodox. "Life begins at creation and is known to have begun at conception," Dr. Byrne commented. He continued: "Death is the event that marks the change from life to non-life or from alive to dead. Death is a state of the absence of life." Only the Creator of life can reverse the "irreversible cessation" or destruction of the heart, lungs, and brain. The last point—resurrection, not resuscitation—is the Christians' hope; without it, the apostle Paul says Christianity is a meaningless religion.

In the 1968 "A Definition of Irreversible Coma," two of Pope Pius XII's 1957 statements were quoted by Dr. Beecher: "…within the competence of the church …But normally one is held to use only ordinary means according to circumstances of persons, places, times, and cultures—that is to say, means that do not involve any grave burden to oneself or another." While Dr. Beecher admitted Pope Pius XII "raised many questions" in his address on "The Prolongation of Life," Dr. Beecher's two conclusions were radically divorced from the Pope's worldview.

Dr. Beecher's twofold conclusion from the quoted comments: (1) the church has no role in determining death. Only a physician can do that. (2) Since this is the case, according to Dr. Beecher, "it's not obligatory [for a physician] to continue extraordinary measures in hopeless cases" (i.e., those cases a physician judges to be hopeless), which circles back to Dr. Beecher's statement in the document that these people *believed* by a physician to be in an "irreversible coma" are a "burden ...on their families, on the hospitals, and on those in need of hospital beds."

Pope Pius XII died in 1958, so he could not respond to Dr. Beecher's interpretation of his comments. It's highly doubtful, however, that he would have endorsed either of his conclusions. Pope Pius XII was a devout Thomistic dualist (more on this below), received aggressive medical treatment for his ailments, and spoke out against the Nazi *Lebenwertes Leben* policies.

During a Christmas radio address in 1942, "The Rights of Man," he addressed the Nazi atrocities head-on:

Are the nations to stand by inactive while this disastrous process goes on? Surely, rather, all men of courage and honor, as they gaze upon the ruins of a social order which has given such tragic proof of its failure to secure the common good, ought to unite in a solemn vow never to rest until valiant souls of every people and every nation of the earth arise in their legions, resolved to bring society back to its immovable center of gravity in the Divine law, and to devote themselves to the service of the human person and of a Divinely ennobled human society. ...Humanity owes this vow to those hundreds of thousands who, without any fault of their own, sometimes only by reason of their nationality or race, are marked down for death or gradual extinction.

Also, in the address to anesthesiologists in 1957, "The Prolongation of Life," which Dr. Beecher conveniently ignored, Pope Pius XII stated the following:

But considerations of a general nature allow us to believe that life continues for as long as its *vital functions* — distinguished from the simple life of organs — manifest themselves *spontaneously or even with the help of artificial processes*. ...In case of insoluble doubt, one must resort to presumtions of law *and of fact*. In general, *it will be necessary to presume that life remains, because there is involved here a fundamental right received from the Creator, and it is necessary to prove with certainty that it has been lost*. ...Public authorities and the laws which concern the use of corpses should, in general, be guided by these same moral and human considerations, since they are based on *human nature itself, which takes precedence over society* in the order of causality and in dignity. In particular, public authorities have the duty to supervise their enforcement and, above all, to take care that a "corpse" *shall not be considered and treated as such until death has been sufficiently proved* (emphasis mine).

Dr. Beecher avoided these points, which deconstruct his social agenda to prove that a non-responsive person with a beating heart, circulation, and aerating lungs (respiration) — vital functions — on a ventilator is a corpse and, therefore, may be plundered for organs or to free up hospital beds to benefit those deemed more worthy to live.

Nevertheless, some Roman Catholics have tried to affirm brain death by focusing on human reason or sentience as a locus of human existence, personhood, and ongoing life. Thomas Aquinas taught: "The light of reason is placed in every man to guide him in his acts." Of course, it's impossible to know how Aquinas would've viewed unresponsive people declared brain dead on a ventilator with a beating heart and aerating lungs since he lived in the thirteenth century. However, there is good evidence that he would have seen these people as alive and humans still bearing God's image.

Patrick Lee and Germain Grisez, philosophy professors at Roman Catholic universities, write in "Total Brain Death: A Reply to Alan Shewmon," *Bioethics*, the following: "We advance a distinct argument for the total brain criterion ...human beings are rational animals — sentient organisms of a specific type—the loss of the radical capacity for sentience (the capacity to sense or to develop the capacity to sense) involves a substantial change, the passing away of the human organism." Thus, when the capacity for sentience (sensation, subjective experience, and feeling), a very elastic and speculative term like irreversibility, is lost, the neurologically impaired person is no longer considered a rational animal or human being.

This view is at odds with traditional Roman Catholic beliefs. First, it assumes philosophical materialism, i.e., the cogitating human brain, the "total brain," is the locus for personhood. This contradicts Thomistic hylomorphism (more on this below). Second, it speculates on the inner workings of a non-responsive person's subjective experiences. The apostle Paul wrote in 1 Corinthians 2:11: "For who knows a person's thoughts except their own spirit within them?" Third, according to this view, the once "rational animal" (a pagan concept from Greek philosophy) is one step lower on the evolutionary ladder and has lost the right to be called a human being created in God's image (more on this below).

Attorney Dennis Horan, the President of Americans Citizens United for Life, was an influential Roman Catholic who jumped on the Dr. Beecher bandwagon and endorsed brain death as death. Horan became the "pro-life" poster boy for UDDA proponents. He was invited to participate in the 1981 Presidential Commission for the Study of Problems in Medicine and Behavioral Research, which published *Defining Death: Medical, Legal, and Ethical Issues in the Determination of Death.*

Before the meeting and drafting of the report, Dr. Byrne met with Dennis Horan. He recalled the difficulty he had trying to arrange a meeting with him. As a dedicated member of Missouri Right to Life, Dr. Byrne spoke to the local chapter president, Ann O'Donnell, and the regional director of the National Right to Life Committee. He thought his dedication to pro-life issues would help set up a meeting, but he was wrong. "Ann had to harass Dennis until he agreed to meet," Dr. Byrne recalled.

Of course, this was no surprise. In 1980, Horan made the following statement in his "Definition of Death an Emerging Consensus," quoted by the

President's Commission verbatim. "Legislation limiting the concept of brain death to [the] cessation of total function of the brain, the brain stem, is beneficial and does not undermine any of the values we seek to support."

The Commission's conclusion:

The views of leaders in the right-to-life movement were also reviewed. In their published statements there is support for the enactment of statutes incorporating total brain death as a basis for determining death. As stated by Dennis Horan President of American Citizens United for Life.

Dr. Byrne recalled his meeting with Horan. "I flew to O'Hare Airport in Chicago and met Dennis. I thought he would take me back to his office. Instead, we had a forty-five-minute lunch at the airport. He ignored what I had to say about brain death not being a true definition of death. He advised me to stop working on the issue of brain death. Dennis suggested that I work on anti-euthanasia activities! He ate, got up, and left me with the bill. I paid the bill and flew back home."

Dr. Byrne continued: "Two doctors known as leaders in the prolife movement were significant advisors to Dennis Horan. Dr. Joseph Stanton, an internist from Boston, and Dr. Eugene Diamond, a pediatrician from Chicago. They were both Roman Catholics and pro-brain death physicians. Joe Stanton was a leading Catholic physician and a medical advisor for American Citizens United for Life. He showed me hospitality once by allowing me to stay at his home in Boston. If I remember correctly, he had a replica statue of the Infant of Prague. I believe his son was a priest in the order of the Jesuits. Dr. Gene Diamond was a Professor of Pediatrics at Loyola University and President of the National Federation of Catholic Physicians' Guilds, now known as the Catholic Medical Association (CMA)."

"Both physicians greatly influenced Dennis Horan and the supposed pro-life acceptance of brain death as death with the President's Commission," Dr. Byrne continued. "It also needs to be said Dennis represented only one pro-life organization among many, and he certainly did not represent the consensus of the pro-life organizations I was affiliated with."

As noted above, the focus on the "light of reason" misunderstands Thomas Aquinas, his belief in hylomorphism, and what the Roman Catholic

Church always taught about the unity of body, soul, and the *imago Dei* that makes a human being a living person. Dr. Byrne explained: "Brain-death criteria are opposed to fundamental teachings in the Roman Catholic Church since the locus of life is not the brain but the unity of soul-body."

In the 1991 Congress on Transplant of Organs, Pope John Paul II stated, "a person can only donate that of which he can deprive himself without serious danger or harm to his own life or personal identity, and for a just and proportionate reason. It is obvious that vital organs can be donated only after death," that is "true death or *mors vera* as understood traditionally in the Roman Catholic Church," added Dr. Byrne.

Pope John Paul II believed the Church should be involved in defining the line between life and death. He also considered the seemingly hopeless cases not as a burden to be eliminated or exploited for organs but as human beings or image bearers of God who merit compassionate care and love until *mors vera*. Pope John Paul's beliefs contradict Dr. Beecher's conclusions about Pope Pius XII's views. Pope John Paul carried on the mantel of papal authority to interpret moral issues facing the modern Roman Catholic Church.

Dr. Doyen Nguyen, a medical doctor, professor of moral theology, and Thomistic theologian, published "Pope John Paul II and the neurological standard for the determination of death: A critical analysis of his address to the Transplantation Society" in a 2017 edition of *The Linacre Quarterly*, and explained the moral and theological underpinnings of the Pope's and Church's teaching:

> The introduction of the "brain death" criterion constitutes a significant paradigm shift in the determination of death. The perception of the public at large is that the Catholic Church has formally endorsed this neurological standard. However, a critical reading of the only magisterial document on this subject, Pope John Paul II's 2000 address, shows that the pope's acceptance of the neurological criterion is conditional in that it entails a twofold requirement. It requires that certain medical presuppositions of the neurological standard are fulfilled, and that its philosophical premise coheres with the Church's teaching on the body-soul union. This article demonstrates that the medical presuppositions are not fulfilled, and that the doctrine of the brain as the central somatic integrator of the body does not cohere either with the current holistic understanding of the human organism or with the Church's Thomistic doctrine of the soul as the form of the body.

Dr. Byrne and his colleagues demonstrated in the 1979 *JAMA* article that the medical presuppositions for a neurological standard of death are seriously flawed. Since his article thirty-eight years ago, the non-scientific assumptions were now glaring, as Dr. Nguyen points out in her 2017 article. Today, no respectable physician equates brain death with the end of a person's biological life.

The first requirement that brain death has a sound scientific and logical basis fails—the second is more dismal for Roman Catholics claiming to be faithful to the Church's doctrine. The neurological criteria assume philosophical materialism, as noted above. The "brain as the central somatic integrator of the body" opposes Thomistic hylomorphism, the official Roman Catholic teaching of a "body-soul union," or "the soul as the form of the body," which is what hylomorphism means.

Dr. Nguyen explains:

First, the pope's teaching on death presupposes Christian anthropology, according to which: (a) the human person is the substantial unity of body and soul, and

(b) the soul is the life principle (substantial form) of the body. This is the doctrine of the Church as taught in the *Catechism* and formally declared by the Council of Vienne in 1312 (CCC, no. 365). Thus, according to Christian anthropology, "the moment of death for each person consists in the definitive loss of the constitutive unity of body and spirit" (John Paul II 2005, no. 4). The death-event, the separation of the soul from the body, brings about "the total disintegration of [the] unitary and integrated whole" (John Paul II 2005, no. 4) that was the person.

According to Roman Catholic teaching, brain death cannot equal death since death is "the total disintegration of [the] unitary and integrated whole" of a person, not merely three pounds of neurological tissue within the skull that *supposedly* serves as the "central somatic integrator of the body."

In 2008, it would have seemed Pope Benedict XVI, the successor of Pope John Paul, would have settled the issue of harvesting organs from "brain dead" donors once and for all for Roman Catholics. In the *Compendium of the Catechism of the Catholic Church*, he made the following declaration:

Individual vital organs cannot be extracted except *ex cadavere*, which, moreover, possesses its own dignity and must be respected. ...The principle criteria of respect for the life of the donator must always prevail so that the extraction of organs be performed only in the case of his/her true death.

The Latin *ex cadavere* means from a corpse, which does not happen for those non-responsive people plundered for organs that have a beating heart, circulation, and respiration. More importantly, "respect for the life of the donator must always prevail" so that organs can only be removed *ex cadavere* after the person changes to a corpse, which can *only* be determined medically and empirically after the heart, lungs, and brain are destroyed. From a doctrinal standpoint, the Roman Catholic Church is in direct opposition to brain death as death.

Next to the 1979 *JAMA* article in importance was the publication of "Brain Death — the Patient, the Physician, and Society" in 1983, which was written in opposition to the 1981 Presidential Commission Report from a medical and legal standpoint. Dr. Byrne co-authored this well-researched document with the two *JAMA* colleagues mentioned earlier and the addition of attorney Peter W. Salsich, Jr., Dean and Professor of Law at St.

Louis University School of Law. The article was published in the *Gonzaga Law Review*.

Although the authors refer to the document as an "article," it is about the size of the book with hundreds of footnotes. It is the work of scholars. Below is the introduction in full (the entire article can be accessed online after performing a title search):

In recent years a radical change has taken place in the practice of medicine, a change still developing yet already grave with consequences both for the interests of each individual and for those of civil society as a whole. The clearest manifestations of this change have clustered around the manner in which it is to be determined that a person has died. From this perspective, the recent and proposed changes in law that have imposed "definitions of death", appear as attempts to have society accept and approve this reorientation of medical practice. What is not so clear is that society has understood the issue sufficiently to have given informed consent.

Though this change in medical practice is more extensive than the particular aspects connected with the determination of death, we must here limit ourselves to this narrower range of problems, which are already sufficiently complex and wide-ranging. We have thought it important to write an article that would present with some fullness the issues which are involved in the new modes of declaring a person dead. All concede the complexity of these issues. Therefore, it is desirable to lay out coherently their intrinsic structure and to state clearly the nodes of interaction between the different disciplines that bear upon them.

Without a comprehensive and carefully structured overview, the different groups with interests in this discussion may continue merely to ignore or rail at one another and to speak rationally only within the limitations of their own group. Part I sets forth the nature and structure of the recent change in medical practice and shows something of its social import. Quite apart from questions of practice, there is a serious theoretical question addressed in Part II: whether the criteria approved by the new statutes are medically correct and properly expressed, and also whether they truly correspond to a person's death. Since one of the major social determinants of law and of its suitability for a given people is their religious and moral convictions, in Part III we seek to find to what extent the new mode of medical practice and the legislation which embodies it are compatible with the major religious traditions of this country. Part IV considers various legal questions not dealt with elsewhere and presents what we regard as the minimum requirements for proper legislation in this domain.

Dr. Byrne's battle to protect and defend life was not over; it had only begun. He would continue his career as a neonatologist and become even more vocal about the "lie of brain death," as Dr. Byrne bluntly puts it. He became a Catholic Medical Association (CMA) member in 1984, and

Dr. Byrne was elevated to the Board of Directors in 1986. In March and September of 1984, Dr. Byrne published two articles in *USA Today*: "Starving Terminal Patients is Murder" and "We Don't Need a Law to Keep Patients Alive" to inform the public of the decline of morals and ethics in medicine.

In 1986, after relocating to Oklahoma, Dr. Byrne accepted Obstetrics & Gynecology and Pediatrics professorships at Oral Roberts University. He was appointed Chairman of the Department of Pediatrics at the same university, an executive committee member, and a member of the Clinical Chair Committee. Eventually, due to his dedication and erudition, Dr. Byrne was elected President of the Medical Faculty Assembly at Oral Roberts University in 1987. He also served as the Medical Director at City of Faith Medical Research in the Department of Newborn Nurseries & Pediatrics and as Chairman of the Ethics Committee.

In 1988, Dr. Byrne was invited to lecture at the Terence Cardinal Cooke Lectureship in New York, and his speech was "Medical, Legal and Ethical Aspects of Brain Death." Moving on into the 1990s, Dr. Byrne published in *The Pharos* "Brain Death—Still a Controversy" (which was translated into German and Italian) and "Reply to Brain Death—the Controversy Continues."

In the Greenhaven Press *Opposing Viewpoint Series*, he published "Brain Death May Not Determine Death." He circulated multiple editions of *Life, Life Support, and Death* for the American Life League. With colleagues, Dr. Byrne published in *Issues in Law and Medicine*: "The Brain Stem in Brain Death" and "Anencephaly—Organ Transplantation?"

Aside from his scholarly labors, Dr. Byrne also wrote to the public. In the *Toledo Blade*, he wrote about the culture of death created by the UDDA and the exploitation of organ donors by the UAGA in a "Declaration of Death Requires Understanding Life," the next chapter's topic.

3

"Declaration of Death Requires Understanding Life"

In the 1990s, Dr. Byrne relocated to his home state of Ohio and accepted the Director of Neonatology position at Riverside Hospital in Toledo. In 1991, he became a staff neonatologist at St. Charles Mercy Hospital in nearby Oregon, Ohio, a position he would hold until 2012.

Dr. Byrne recalled the opposition as he continued defending life from conception until death. "Shirley often reminded me, 'Remember, Paul, you must keep your job.' I did the brain death work but kept it in the background as much as possible." Nevertheless, the Holy Spirit kept prompting Dr. Byrne. In 1994, he was compelled to write an article for public consumption in *The Toledo Blade*.

The article "Declaration of Death Requires Understanding Life" pulled together Dr. Byrne's expertise as a neonatologist to explain the beginning of life and his passion for confronting the lie about brain death to define the end of life. It declared the moral imperative all humans share to protect the most vulnerable people among us.

When we open our morning paper and see a photo of a young man whose life was saved by an organ transplant, our natural sympathies are evoked almost subliminally.

When we turn on the evening news and hear the plaintive plea of distraught parents, begging for the "gift of life" for their little girl, our critical faculties are somnambulant.

Yet ethical and reasoned life requires that we form critical judgments that take into account substantive distinctions. A vital—literally vital—distinction is the difference between the *donation* of paired and unpaired organs.

Thinking motivated solely by feelings tends to drive people into immoral or harmful acts, so laws are enacted to promote a reasonable course of action to prevent injury and to uphold a moral standard. For example, a father motivated by deep feelings may want to donate his heart—an unpaired organ—to a daughter with end-stage heart failure. The law, however, forbids this lethal act to the father, even though it is the father's selfless desire to donate his heart to save his daughter's life.

What is not reasonable are laws like the Uniform Determination of Death Act (UDDA) that permit murderous acts by harvesting vital organs from living donors declared dead by a neurological standard. The feelings motivating this lethal act align with our empathy for those needing a life-saving organ. Still, it's at the expense of another person's life. Ultimately, laws that permit ending the life of another person for utilitarian purposes are the same as the *Lebensunwertes Leben* policies in Nazi Germany.

Dr. Byrne moves on in the article to discuss what constitutes the life and death of a human being:

The ongoing life of an organism as complex as a human being requires the interdependence of organs and systems to maintain the unity of the body. A system is a group of organs, tissues, and cells organized in a particular manner to carry out specific functions of the body. The human body encompasses many systems, including major systems that are essential to the continuation of physical life.

The circulatory system, which includes the heart, is an example of a vital system. Without the structure and functioning of the circulatory system, with or without external assistance, life will end. The respiratory system, which includes the lungs and trachea (windpipe), is another vital system. A ventilator — commonly, but not accurately called a respirator — may be required to support, not supplant, respiration: It is the man, not the machine, who breathes, after all.

The central nervous system, which includes the brain, is yet another major system. The brain comprises many parts that function interdependently, just as the brain operates interdependently with organs and systems to maintain the oneness of the body. No single organ or system dominates the body. Cooperation, not control, is key to preserving the unity vital to life's continuance.

What then of death? Death signifies the end of life on earth for a unique, irreplaceable person. Death can be described in terms of biology and biochemistry, basic sciences studied by every physician.

Life support is a terrible term. It leads people to believe the "unique, irreplaceable person" requiring medical and mechanical assistance is dead — the person's death is masked by life support — but this is incorrect. The term "life support" promotes the idea that if all the medical apparatus is removed, the person's heart will immediately stop beating, breathing will cease, and masked blueness, coldness, and stiffness will be revealed.

The reality is a pacemaker, ventilator, and medications require a still-living heart, lungs, liver, kidneys, and brain to work. These same living organs are also needed for successful transplant surgeries. The interdependent cooperation of circulatory, respiratory, and neurological systems and anatomy down to physiological processes and cells controls a person's physical life. Death ought not to be declared unless these three systems, at a minimum, are destroyed.

"After the destruction of these three systems, then death can be declared from a medical standpoint. 'True death' has arrived," Dr. Byrne declared with a note of solemnity. Life support is also exposed for what it cannot do—resurrect a dead person to life. The difference is between maintaining an ongoing life and not "life support" to keep a corpse alive—a crucial distinction, indeed, especially for Christians who affirm a belief in "the resurrection of the body," as the Apostle Creed states.

Dr. Byrne continues:

There are facts of life and realities of death. Under Hippocratic medicine, it was the physician's awesome responsibility not to declare a person "dead" while he was yet alive. No one was pronounced dead unless and until the heart had ceased to beat, there was no evidence of any breathing, and no response of any kind from the central nervous system.

In the past, the physician took the time needed to determine death because he did not wish to treat the living as dead. Today, however, death is often declared in a rush to judgment lest we treat the "brain dead" as alive. How did this change occur, and why?

He then mentions the 1968 Harvard report and the move to redefine death with neurological criteria. "Conveniently," Dr. Byrne comments in the article, "newly coined 'brain death' allowed the 'harvesting' of vital organs, thus aiding and abetting the growing practice of organ transplantation."

The excising of a beating heart would have constituted murder under traditional standards for determining death. The fact remains that brain death and death are neither identical nor equivalent. If they were, there would be no need for different terms.

Another crucial distinction that is often

overlooked! Why do we need two definitions to determine the single event of death? Dr. Byrne concludes: "The physician has a moral duty and a professional responsibility not to pronounce someone dead while he is yet alive," and adds:

Death cannot be determined and should not be declared unless there is no doubt whatsoever that life on earth had ended for the person declared dead. Any doubt must always be resolved in favor of life, and the law should be written to protect the lives of every citizen including those from whom a vital organ is about to be taken.

Human life is an endowment from the Creator of life. Therefore, every person possesses unalienable rights, and fundamental is the "right to life," regardless of how people feel, what the majority endorses, and a person's mental state. Most of the German nation embraced the *Lebensunwertes Leben* policies of Hitler to euthanize the mentally disabled for utilitarian purposes. This ugly historical fact of human behavior should cause Americans to pause and reflect.

The lives of everyone should be protected by laws that the Constitution underwrites, and presently, laws in the United States (US) conflict with the Constitution, harm vulnerable people, and uphold immoral acts. Each person the Creator creates is a unique, unrepeatable, and irreplaceable human being from conception until the end of biological life. Life is life, and the Creator of life expects his dependent creatures to protect and preserve it until death is unavoidable.

"At the moment of conception," Dr. Byrne explained during our interview, "the person is manifest. Conception occurs within the mother's body when the baby can be identified at the one-cell stage known as conceptus. In the conceptus, the new person's genetic material is present. Now, the invisible is visible. Conception is the manifestation of our earthly existence. The beginning of every person is a creation of God. Human life on the earth is a substantial fact of the unity of soul and body. The new person is unique and unrepeatable."

While the parents and child share similar DNA, a dissimilarity in the God-given spirit (distinctive personal identity) in union with the body makes the baby different from his or her parents. The baby's DNA has either XX (female) or XY (male) chromosomes, which means the new person's gender is fixed. "The true beginning of life on earth occurs at conception," Dr. Byrne stated. "Then, in about six to seven days after conception, the developing baby attaches to the mother's uterus, which is referred to as implantation."

"Incidentally," Dr. Byrne said, "birth control pills like Depo-Provera, Norplant, 'the patch,' and Intra-Uterine Devices injure the inner lining of the mother's uterus, making it unsuitable for implantation to begin or to be sustained." Notice that the baby's life started before implantation into the mother's uterus, so these pills and devices kill the baby. "Thus," Dr. Byrne exclaimed, "these are abortifacients. Some have based their use of these agents on the false assumption that life does not begin until implantation, but they are wrong. The truth is that medical and scientific facts indicate that the life of a new, unique person is present at conception, and implantation is a stage in the embryonic process."

Dr. Byrne continued: "The life of a human on earth is a continuum from conception until true death. For life on the earth to continue inside and outside the mother's womb, each person must take in oxygen, water, and nutrients" and remove waste products. The implantation stage sets into motion a process of embryogenesis in the mother. At this time, the baby's anatomy develops, and physiological processes begin so the baby will be prepared for a life outside the womb.

Eventually, "cells, tissues, organs, and systems interdependently function to maintain the unity of the body, which is a soul-body unity, a life-body unity," Dr. Byrne commented. All humans are dependent beings from conception until death. Those who declare people dead with a beating heart, who require a ventilator's inspiratory action, overlook their *own* moment-by-moment dependency on the creation and other people to survive.

"Ventilation and respiration are required for life on the earth," Dr. Byrne continued. "Ventilation is the movement of air; respiration is the exchange of oxygen and carbon dioxide in the lungs and via the circulation in all the body's tissues." Dr. Byrne produced a pamphlet he created for the American Life League, *To Breathe is To Live: The Ventilator Assists Breathing*, and pointed out the following passage:

In everyday life, for breathing to occur, an impulse originates in the brain and is conducted along nerves to muscles used in breathing. These muscles are those of the chest wall and the diaphragm (a muscle that separates the chest from the abdomen). The muscles contract, causing the chest to expand, resulting in lungs filled with oxygen-rich air. Nerve impulses stop and the muscles relax. The chest elastically recoils, exhaling carbon dioxide into the air. Other organs used in breathing include the trachea (the windpipe), smaller air passages known as the bronchi and bronchioles, and the lungs.

Oxygen and carbon dioxide exchange occur in the lungs and living tissues throughout the body via circulation. The heart pumps, circulating blood to and through the lungs and then throughout the body. In the lungs, the blood takes in oxygen and gives up carbon dioxide. Then the blood circulates throughout the rest of the body where an opposite exchange occurs: the blood gives up oxygen and takes in carbon dioxide. This exchange in the lungs and in the tissues is respiration.

"On the other hand," Dr. Byrne resumed, "heartbeat is intrinsic to the heart. The heart has nerves that cause the heart muscle to contract and stop contracting. The heart beats without impulses from the brain. No organ, including the brain, controls the other organs. The respiratory, circulatory, and central nervous systems are vital.

Without the functioning activities of these three vital systems, life on earth ends quickly."

"Without respiration and circulation," Dr. Byrne continued, "the person's health deteriorates, and death will occur unless breathing and circulation are restored quickly." He produced the pamphlet mentioned above once again and pointed out the paragraphs below:

Sometimes breathing needs assistance, e.g., an inhaler or a ventilator. Experience shows that an inhaler can be helpful for asthma. A ventilator can be beneficial to treat other diseases and injuries. While we are grateful for the ability to breathe without the need of an inhaler or ventilator, if ever these are needed to assist breathing, we should request them and treatment with them ought to be expected.

When the parts of the brain that control breathing or the organs and tissues for breathing are diseased or injured, a ventilator helps until normal functioning is restored. For example, people with head injuries and respiratory diseases typically receive relief and help from the use of a ventilator.

This machine is properly called a "ventilator" since it supports the ventilation part of breathing. In other words, a ventilator moves air; it does not and cannot cause the other part of breathing—respiration. That is, it does not and cannot exchange oxygen and carbon dioxide as occurs in lungs and body tissues. Respiration can only happen when the body's respiratory and circulatory systems are otherwise intact and functioning properly. Respiration is a human function, not a machine's. The more accurate term "ventilator" should always be used.

The ventilator moves air into air spaces to help the patient to breathe more effectively. The ventilator does not move the air out. Elastic recoil of the lungs and chest moves the air out of the patient. A ventilator can be effective as support of respiration only in a living patient, never in a corpse.

When the living body of a person with interdependence of organs and systems receives an adequate supply of needed oxygen, and carbon dioxide is exhaled, healing can occur. If respiration is not supported adequately by the ventilator, although all other treatments remain in place, death nevertheless can occur.

By now it should be clear that in terms of function, a ventilator, like an inhaler, is a means of treatment for a patient who needs help breathing.

Dr. Byrne looked me in the eye and said: "The important thing to know is that both the ventilator and the inhaler are forms of treatment. Therefore, the decision to use a ventilator should be made in the same way decisions about other forms of treatment and care are made — by determining whether it will protect and preserve life."

Again, we are reminded that we are all dependent people, and there are modern treatments and equipment that can be an effective means to preserve life and prevent human suffering. Who would snatch an inhaler out of the hand of an asthmatic when an attack strikes? The person who denies a rescue inhaler to a person with an asthma attack is oblivious to his or her moment-by-moment dependency on air to breathe.

Nevertheless, physicians in intensive care units (ICUs) who take a solemn oath not to harm the people under their care engage in this type of behavior when they perform the apnea test to declare brain death. During this exam, the ventilator is stopped "sometimes for up to ten minutes, and the patient is suffocated," Dr. Byrne exclaimed, "and it is even performed repeatedly on people with head injuries!" These cruel medical doctors violate their solemn oath and, worse, they disconnect the ventilator for up to ten minutes, which deprives the patient of roughly 160-200 cycles of ventilation during the apnea test.

"Without respiration and circulation," Dr. Byrne reiterated, "health of the person deteriorates, and death will occur unless breathing and circulation are restored quickly. This deterioration manifests in the cessation of vital activities, and then in disintegration, dissolution, lysis, destruction, corruption, decay, and putrefaction of cells and tissues of organs and systems." There is an actual line between life and death. "For justice to protect living persons," Dr. Byrne continued, "no one ought to be declared dead unless respiratory and circulatory systems and the entire brain have been destroyed."

"The moment of separation of the soul from the body is the moment of true death," which, in Latin, Dr. Byrne noted is "*mors vera*." He said: "Doctors are accustomed to noting the 'time of death,' but the exact moment of this separation, which is true death, cannot be detected. Only the observation that it has already definitely occurred can. After the end of biological life, the body does not respond and has significantly changed. After death, these pathologic changes continue. They cannot be stopped."

There is a reason for the term dead weight. When the soul, spirit, or immaterial life force no longer animates the body, these people become lifeless and inert. Dr. Byrne concluded: "Life and death cannot exist simultaneously in the same person. People are not truly dead when there is respiration, circulation, and a beating heart."

Even with pushback from colleagues, it appeared Dr. Byrne was progressing on the national and international fronts with his pro-life commitments. In 1995, he was promoted to vice president at the Catholic Medical Association (CMA), formerly the National Federation of Catholic Physicians Guilds (NFCPG). The following year, he became the president-elect and, in 1997, served a designated one-year term as the organization's president. In 1997, with Dr. Byrne at the helm, the NFCPG became the CMA. During the same year, Dr. Byrne served as the Chairman for the 1997 sixty-sixth annual CMA conference, which had the theme of "Morals or Ethics?"

The CMA's journal, *The Linacre Quarterly*, which was already referenced, is an essential scholarly publication of the medical group. The name was chosen to honor Thomas Linacre, a physician and priest in sixteenth-century England. According to the CMA website, "Dr. Linacre served as the private physician to King Henry VIII and was a founding member of the Royal College of Physicians. He was well known for his scholarship, high standards for scientific medicine, and strong Catholic faith."

Dr. Byrne had a flurry of publications in *The Linacre Quarterly* from 1997 until 1999. Of note for this book are: "Quinlan Re-Examined," "Life, Life Support, and Death: Principles, Guidelines, Policies and Procedures for Making Decisions that Respect Life," and "Brain Death is False." During these years, Dr. Byrne continued his professorship as a Clinical Professor of Pediatrics at the University of Toledo College of Medicine, a position he has held since 1996.

His academic labors continued inside and outside the church. In 1999, in collaboration with the world-renowned pediatric neurologist Dr. D. Alan Shewmon, Dr. Byrne published "Consciousness in Congenitally Decorticate Children: Developmental Vegetative State as Self-Fulling Prophecy," *Developmental Medicine & Child Neurology*. The abstract for the article states:

According to traditional neurophysiological theory, consciousness requires neocortical functioning, and children born without cerebral hemispheres necessarily remain indefinitely in a developmental vegetative state. Four children between 5 and 17 years old are reported with congenital brain malformations involving total or near-total absence of cerebral cortex but who, nevertheless, possessed discriminative awareness: for example, distinguishing familiar from unfamiliar people and environments, social interaction, functional vision, orienting, musical preferences, appropriate affective responses, and associative learning.

Traditional neurology theorists believe consciousness is found in the uppermost layer of the brain or the neocortex, as Dr. Harvey Sarnat affirmed in the first chapter. However, the children in this study had "total or near-total absence of cerebral cortex." Nevertheless, they could still interact with the environment around them, which violated the "neocortical functioning" dogma. This widely held assumption, which gained the status of a neurological fact of brain function about subjective experience, was untrue, not just by one or two patients but several.

TK lived twenty years after a "brain death" diagnosis. TK was born in 1979, and after he turned four, he contracted bacterial meningitis due to Haemophilus influenza. As a result, TK had a rise in intracranial pressure, temperature problems, and increased urine output that caused electrolyte imbalances. Hypovolemia with low blood pressure followed, further exacerbating TK's brain injury. Serial electroencephalograms (EEGs) revealed he had no electrical activity in the brain.

He ended up in a coma at Bergan Mercy Hospital, Nebraska, and Dr. Byrne treated TK while covering for a colleague. Dr. Byrne recalled his involvement with TK. "There he was, lying in a crib in the hospital with his mother sitting by his side. I told his mother, 'The nurse called me because Todd's blood pressure is low.' I said, 'I can prescribe medications to raise his blood pressure,' and asked her what she wanted me to do. Instantly, TK's mother looked at me and said: 'Well, get on with it!' I ordered the nurse to administer a dopamine infusion, which elevated his blood pressure and stabilized his vital signs."

Eventually, TK was discharged home under the loving care of his mother on a portable ventilator with a gastrostomy tube (G-tube) for feeding and administering medications, which is commonly referred to as a feeding tube. Throughout the rest of his life, TK only required basic nursing care, which his mother provided and found meaningful. He did not need future intervention for critical instability. He died in 2004 from a cardiac arrest.

TK's mother consented to have an autopsy of his brain, and the findings completely and comprehensibly destroyed the UDDA concept of total-brain death as death and challenged the traditional assumptions made by the neurologists mentioned above. Before the autopsy, a computer tomography (CT) scan demonstrated calcification or hardening throughout TK's brain. Magnetic resonance imaging (MRI) revealed no identifiable anatomical brain structures, and the autopsy supported these diagnostic findings.

After TK's skull was sawed apart, there was only a hard four-inch walnut-like tissue mass. The visual inspection of the pathologist performing the autopsy confirmed the MRI finding—no brain structures were present. Sectioning by a saw of the rock-like mass confirmed the CT findings. The microscopic examination of these sections revealed mineralized deposits that appeared "mummified," the pathologist reported. There were no recognizable nerve structures, cells, or specific neuronal markers to indicate the *remote possibility of brain function*.

Yet, TK lived at home for two decades on a

portable ventilator with a feeding tube under the care of his devoted mother. The significance of TK's life and the persistence of a mother caring for her son cannot be underestimated. TK single-handedly exposed the fallacy of the UDDA neurological standard and put the "experts" to shame. He forced physicians, philosophers, and theologians to change their understanding of brain death or to embrace the Nazi "life unworthy of life" doctrine as it relates to ending the lives of vulnerable people like TK.

Many, even up until now, opt for the latter — just like the hordes who clung to the murderous policies of Hitler. The Nazi *Lebensunwertes Leben* minions euthanized five thousand children born with genetic deficits and 200,000 human beings with neurocognitive problems. Some, like Dr. Shewmon, however, were humbler, more compassionate, and willing to be honest with themselves and the facts of life. The lives of TK and the other children in the collaborative article brought Dr. Shewmon and Dr. Byrne together in more ways than one. Until the present day, their forces are now united against the UDDA neurological definition of death.

In 2000, Dr. Byrne was promoted to the Director of Neonatology at St. Charles Mercy Hospital. Shortly after that, he published with colleagues the scholarly works *Beyond Brain Death: The Case Against Brain Based Criteria for Human Death* and *Brain Death and Disorders of Consciousness: Proceedings of the Fourth International Symposium on Coma and Death* (Kluwer Academic Publishers). In the 2001 and 2005 editions of the *Catholic World Report*, Dr. Byrne published "Are Organ Transplants Ever Licit?" and "'Brain Death' is not Death," which led to an invitation to present at the Pontifical Academy of Sciences, Vatican City, Italy.

At the Pontifical Academy of Sciences in February of 2005, he lectured about "Signs of Death." Nine months later, Dr. Byrne was invited back to Italy to present "Death—The Absence of Life" to the Research Council of Italy. The result of the presentation was the publication of *Finis Vitae: Is "Brain Death" True Death?* in 2006. Then, in 2009 and 2012, in Rome, Italy, he organized and presented "Signs of Life, Is 'Brain Death' Still Life?" and at the International Congress, "The Boundaries of the Human, the Human Being at the Time of the Biotechnological Revolution." In the meantime, Dr. Byrne's tireless pro-life labors would continue in America with the establishment of the Life Guardian Foundation in 2009 and as a guest columnist for *Renew America*.

Dr. Byrne started to write articles for *Renew America* in 2007. His first piece was "Vital Distinctions in Transplantation," and all his essays follow his life mission to be a defender of life. These articles, spanning sixteen years, may be categorized in the following way: medical ethics from a traditional Christian perspective surrounding the subject of organ donation and transplants, issues relating to the definition of life and death, and the obligations of the Church and State to advocate for God-created life and the constitutional rights and liberties of Americans. Many of these topics overlap in a single piece but can be grouped topically. Dr. Byrne's writing for *Renew America* is a ministry of the Life Guardian Foundation, and his most engaging articles chronicle his activity as a private physician and patient advocate.

In 2013, Dr. Byrne became involved in the case of Jahi McMath, a twelve-year-old girl from

California, who made national and international news after being declared brain-dead on December 12, 2013. The teen had her tonsils and adenoids surgically removed at Children's Hospital Oakland to treat sleep apnea. She developed postoperative bleeding and had a cardiac arrest. Jahi was resuscitated and required a ventilator to breathe. According to her doctors, the loss of circulation caused brain death. Her mother, Nailah, refused to accept that she was dead, and a legal battle ensued. Dr. Byrne defended Jahi's life and eventually prescribed treatment for her.

Dr. Byrne recalled when he first arrived at Children's Hospital Oakland: "Initially, I was not permitted access by hospital security. Jahi's stepfather, however, aware of my arrival, came out to greet me. With a look of relief on his face, he said, 'Thank God you're here, pastor.' I was then permitted access to Jahi." Dr. Byrne provided professional medical advocacy and help to Jahi and her family.

After a legal battle that interfered with adequate treatment for Jahi, she was released by the hospital and transported to St. Peter's University Hospital, New Brunswick, New Jersey. State law in New Jersey allows families to reject a brain death diagnosis if it conflicts with their religious beliefs. Eventually, Jahi was moved to an apartment on a portable ventilator and had a feeding tube. Dr. Byrne chronicled the events, treatment, and reflections on the *Renew America* website, which will be reproduced in collaboration with Dr. Byrne.

Dr. Byrne's first article, "Jahi is NOT Truly Dead, Wesley Smith," was published on December 24, 2013, two weeks after her diagnosis of brain death. The piece was in response to Smith's article: "'Brain Dead' Term Too Loosely Used," published by the *National Review* on December 19.

Wesley J. Smith, a senior fellow at the Discovery Institute's Center on Human Exceptionalism, consults for the Patient's Rights Council. He is an influential voice in Roman Catholic circles. Dr. Byrne takes issue with two assertions made by Smith: (1) brain-dead people are "functionally decapitated" and, therefore, dead, and (2) there needs to be a uniform consensus among the different states to affirm this view of death. Dr. Byrne sets up an answer-and-response dialogue between Smith and himself in the argumentative style reminiscent of Thomas Aquinas.

Smith writes:

> In Jahi's case, brain dead actually means a declaration of *"death by neurological criteria,"* one of the two legal methods for declaring the bona fide death of a human being. To be declared dead by neurological criteria does not mean there are no brain cells remaining alive. Rather, it means that medical tests, observation of the patient post injury, and history of the case demonstrate that the patient's *brain and each of its constituent parts have irreversibly ceased to function as a brain.* As one doctor told me, it is as if the patient was functionally decapitated. ...A huge problem in this field is that there are no uniform criteria for declaring death by neurological criteria, with testing requirements varying from state to state, and in some instances, hospital to hospital. That needs to change.

As noted earlier, function or non-function does not equal existence and life; function and non-function correspond to conditions of activity or idleness, not a state of being. Functional decapitation is patently absurd, and it is equally foolish to create a uniform law based on this nonsense.

Smith asserts, "To be declared dead by neurological criteria does not mean there are no brain cells remaining alive."

Dr. Byrne replies, "Oh really? Would that be

like a little bit pregnant? The language of the Uniform Determination of Death (UDDA) is 'irreversible cessation of all functions of the entire brain, including the brain stem,' and it means just that. It means no brain cells are alive, and because of this, the *entire brain*, including the brain stem, has ceased to function to promote ongoing life." People like Smith use the term brain death too loosely, and they are so loose with their definition that they violate the UDDA requirement for brain death!

"So," Dr. Byrne exclaims, "Wesley, are you writing that Jahi has or could have living brain cells? Do you have to be a clever writer to conclude that 'all' and 'entire' and 'including the brain stem' does not mean no brain cells remain alive? If this is what it does not mean, what do all and entire and including mean?" If Jahi has brain cells "remaining alive," then she is not dead according to the UDDA, "*all functions* of the *entire brain, including the brain stem*" (emphasis mine).

The reality is Jahi still has the function of neurons, dendrites, synapses, ionic exchange, secretion and absorption of neurotransmitters, neural networks, microvascular circulation, neuronal and hormonal secretion, and who knows what else!

Smith, "Rather, it means that medical tests, observation of the patient post injury, and history of the case demonstrate that the patient's brain and each of its constituent parts have irreversibly ceased to function as a brain."

Dr. Byrne responds, "How can you come to this conclusion? What does 'irreversible cessation of *all* functions of the *entire* brain' mean if some cellular parts of the brain are admittedly still alive? Wesley, your answer to explain how some parts of the brain can remain alive and a person can still be dead is absurd. You write, 'As one doctor told me, it is as if the patient was functionally decapitated.' That one doctor and you have a misconception about decapitation!"

"Decapitation is what the Guillotine does. The result of this traumatic event is the irreversible cessation of brain function by severing the head from the body. Decapitation is undoubtedly not the case for people like Jahi, who has vital systems functioning in her body to cause a heartbeat, respiration, circulation, excretion of waste products, infection resistance, blood pressure regulation, temperature fluctuations, and healing. Her body's ongoing integration of biological systems indicates there may still be brain and body communication. So, the brain has not necessarily 'ceased to function as a brain' in people meeting your standard of 'functionally decapitated.'"

Jahi taught the medical community some important lessons during the seventeen years of her life because while she was "functionally decapitated" for four years, dead in Smith's view, she experienced new neuronal growth, neuroplasticity, and the recovery of some higher brain functions. Jahi was alive! She was misdiagnosed as dead, which is not uncommon for people in her condition.

Advances in modern neuroscience also warrant caution when speculating about another person's mental state when he or she still has vital bodily functions. Since the discovery of a "persistent vegetative state" (PVS) made by Dr. Fred Plum in 1972, he later found that the condition was not always permanent. In some cases, it could be reversed. *Nature* published an article in 2000 showing evidence of damaged neurons regenerating in the central nervous system. Also, new neural networks may form through neuroplasticity to promote compensatory mechanisms in the brain. A 1996 *British Medical Journal* (*BMJ*) study found that seventeen of forty participants considered vegetative were misdiagnosed, and one-third experienced recovery during the research period.

It is also a well-known medical fact that after head trauma and oxygen deprivation, time to decrease intracranial swelling and utilizing neuroprotective strategies can foster healing in the brain. Jahi was denied this essential treatment. "After all," Dr. Byrne continues, "according to Wesley, she is 'functionally decapitated.' Sadly, Jahi would've received better care to preserve her organs than to treat her medical problems if her mother had consented to organ donation and accepted the death diagnosis."

Wesley continues, "A huge problem in this field is that there are no uniform criteria for declaring death by neurological criteria, with testing requirements varying from state to state, and in some instances, hospital to hospital. That needs to change."

Dr. Byrne replies, "It is controversial because thirty disparate sets of criteria were published between 1968 and 1978 and as recently as 2008. Also, a survey by leading neurologists in the US indicated no consensus on which criteria should be used. Yes, dead by one, but alive by other criteria in different states."

"Further, in 2010, it was reported that neurological criteria are not even 'evidence-based,' as 'functional decapitation' assumes, which means they are not based on scientific studies. Which criteria can be acceptable? How about the loss of cardiopulmonary function to determine the loss of life? Or how about an actual decapitation or crushing of the head?"

Dr. Byrne continues tongue-in-cheek, "Here comes Wesley on his white horse; he's going to straighten all this brain death-as-death stuff out. He now agrees that there are 'no uniform criteria' for a declaration of 'brain death.' Then, he provides the answer, 'This needs to change.' The one physician he looked to suggested 'functional decapitation' as the needed change, and that's good enough for Smith, too."

"Wesley is correct," Dr. Byrne continues,

"change is needed, but it must be changed to protect and preserve life until true death. Let's start the change by informing the public that when you answer 'yes' at the DMV to be an organ donor, you have agreed to have your heart and other vital organs cut out of you before you're dead. Who would become a registered organ donor if they knew this truth?"

"The need for 'brain death' is, and has always been from its onset, Wesley, a move to eliminate the 'controversy' about cutting out the heart and other healthy perfused organs from uninformed registered organ donors. A person with a beating heart, circulation, and respiration from whom organs are taken for transplantation is not a corpse or in a state of 'functional decapitation' — the person is still alive!"

"You then write, 'Many bioethicists — of the type who once assured a wary public that brain dead was truly dead — agree, but because they want access to the organs of patients with clearly working brains, such as a patient diagnosed as unconscious but who can breathe without medical assistance.' Wait! 'Functionally decapitated' brains with cells 'remaining alive' are technically still working, so these people have not experienced irreversible cessation. They are, in fact, 'patients with clearly working brains.' You are contradicting yourself, Wesley!"

"More egregiously," Dr. Byrne exclaims, "you write: 'Under the law, brain dead is 'dead' when it connotes death by neurological criteria. In such circumstances, if accurately determined, there is no legal right to continue life support of what is, essentially, a corpse.' A corpse does not have a beating heart, circulation, or respiration! Nor does it excrete waste products, mature, heal wounds, deliver babies, have blood pressure variations in response to stress, or require paralyzing agents when the body moves during an organ-harvest surgery."

"All these functions have occurred in people 'functionally decapitated' with brain cells 'remaining alive,' including Jahi, who requires a ventilator and a feeding tube. You dare call Jahi a corpse whose dead condition is masked by life support. Shame on you, Wesley!"

On January 14, 2014, roughly one year after Jahi was declared dead at Children's Hospital Oakland but was now thriving in a cozy apartment in New Jersey, Dr. Byrne published "Jahi McMath is a Living Person." As the weeks and months passed, Jahi started to show signs of responsiveness, finally catching Dr. Shewmon's attention.

Dr. Shewmon watched video footage and observed her personally for six hours. He also noticed that an MRI scan nine months after her brain injury indicated the brain's higher regions were preserved, so much for being "functionally decapitated." Dr. Shewmon determined that Jahi was in a Minimally Conscious State (MCS) and testified the same before the California Superior Court, which meant she had a level of awareness.

One year after the tragic event, "the neurologist Calixto Machado studied the heart rate of Jahi McMath and found that it was environmentally responsive—this responsiveness being a clear brainstem function," reported Dr. Shewmon. Jahi had brain function in her cortex (higher brain) and showed signs of recovery in her severely damaged brainstem (lower brain). Shortly after that, Jahi also started to respond to verbal commands to move.

Dr. Shewmon determined these movements

were too complex to be reflexes. He noted further that Jahi went through puberty and started menstruating, which requires a functioning hypothalamus (part of the brain). He concluded at the time of her declaration of death, the bedside neurological examinations, EEGs, and cerebral blood flow studies (CTs and MRIs) could not detect the level of life she possessed.

Dr. Byrne's article from *Renew America* is reproduced below, with editing and additional reflections from him.

Jahi is a living person and has been a live person on earth since her conception inside her mother's womb. Jahi's heart beats 100,000 times daily, a typical rate for most people. Her heartbeat is initiated in her heart, just like yours and mine. Jahi's pulse and blood pressure are regular and forceful. Jahi digests her food, urinates, and has bowel movements like everyone else. Jahi's temperature is 98 degrees Fahrenheit, and her favorite blanket is tucked around her for comfort. Her metabolism is working fine. Jahi is on a ventilator, which only pushes air into her lungs, but Jahi forces the air out.

I have been at the bedside of Jahi, and she is not dead. Those who claim Jahi is dead are not using common sense and are discriminating against the mentally disabled. Jahi has serious problems, but she is not dead. Why does Jahi have to prove she is living? Do you have to prove that you are living? The Congress of Neurological Surgeons (CNS) declared that Jahi was dead because she had "a complete lack of blood flow to the brain [and the] absence of any electrical activity." Then why is her body doing many things everyone else's body does? There have been cases where people have had no detectable blood flow in the brain or electrical activity but have fully recovered. Why not this teenager who is still growing? What is different about Jahi? Shouldn't she be given the benefit of the doubt? The extensive high-tech medical testing interpreted by the experts was not good enough to detect the level of life Jahi possessed (an awful thought to consider since many people are declared dead every day with low-tech bedside testing by run-of-the-mill doctors).

The CNS article also includes the "absence of cranial nerve response" concerning Jahi. Only a few, not all, reflexes of the brainstem are tested when brain death is declared. Let's get that straight. An example of the difference between a reflex and a function is found in the leg. When the knee is tapped with a reflex hammer, it jumps. The function of the leg, however, is its ability to walk, which the hammer-to-knee reflex does not elicit. Several other reflexes and prior functions cause the function of walking. The only function of the brainstem that is evaluated is the ability of the patient to breathe, which is not as straightforward as it seems.

A ventilator supports the vital inspiratory activity of Jahi's breathing, but over time, this could change — it has with many others — especially in a young girl who is still growing. The way the brainstem reflex is tested for the function of breathing is the cruel and harmful apnea test. Physicians performed the apnea test three times on Jahi, and the ventilator was stopped for ten minutes each time. Try holding your breath for one minute, never mind ten! During that time, carbon dioxide increased in Jahi's brain, and the result was additional swelling, injury, and trauma to her already oxygen-deprived brain. God only knows what this would do to a brainstem reflex.

While at Children's Hospital Oakland and during the court litigation to continue her care, Jahi was starved for thirty days and denied a tracheostomy and feeding tube. She was only provided intravenous water, sugar, and salt but was refused vitamins, minerals, proteins, and lipids to foster nervous tissue healing and meet her nutritional requirements. Jahi needed the tracheostomy to be treated outside Children's Hospital Oakland, but she was also denied that.

Jahi is alive with a beating heart, blood pressure, pulse, and respiration, albeit on a ventilator with a feeding tube. Now, Jahi is confounding the death-dealing elites in California, who ignore their dependency on air, food, and other people to survive, who, with high-brow hubris, revile those less fortunate than them. By God's grace, Jahi is healing, recovering, and responding to the outside world — she is doing things corpses don't do.

On January 18, 2014, Dr. Byrne published "Jahi McMath's Functioning Hypothalamus: Some Social and Scientific Considerations." Below, the author, Christopher W. Bogosh (CWB), discussed the article with Dr. Paul A. Byrne (PAB).

CWB: "Jahi McMath's Functioning Hypothalamus: Some Social and Scientific Considerations" raises important matters about justice and the scientific application of the neurological criteria of the UDDA. How would you describe the core issues?

PAB: Whatever our biases about Jahi McMath's "brain-death" diagnosis, we ought to consider the responsibilities of taking sides in this controversy and the potential implications for society. A vital component of the McMath debate has, for the most part, been ignored in public dialogue. She fulfilled the AAN Guidelines for brain death but not the UDDA requirement for declaration of death by neurological criteria requiring "irreversible cessation of all functions of the entire brain," as evidenced by the ongoing function of Jahi's hypothalamus.

CWB: What is the hypothalamus?

PAB: The hypothalamus is a part of the brain linked to the pituitary gland. The pituitary gland produces hormones after it receives signals from the hypothalamus. It's the main link between the endocrine and nervous systems. It is crucial in maintaining brain-body balance, a process called homeostasis.

The hypothalamus receives chemical messages from nerve cells in the brain and nerve cells in the body. It also responds to sensory stimuli from outside the body to produce various hormones or chemical messages to communicate with endogenous glands in the brain or body. The hypothalamus is involved in body temperature, blood pressure, heart rate, breathing, hunger and thirst, mood, sex drive, and sleep.

CWB: Why did the Children's Hospital Oakland physicians and the specialist appointed by the California Superior Court think Jahi's hypothalamus stopped functioning?

PAB: Jahi was not self-regulating her body temperature for most of December, which indicated a sign of lost hypothalamic function. On December 24, 2013, California Superior Court Justice Judge Grillo ruled that McMath was legally dead according to the UDDA neurological standard. He based his decision on the medical evidence presented by physicians and an independent expert from Children's Hospital Oakland.

The judge ruled, however, to require the hospital to continue mechanical ventilation until

December 30, 2013, and extended the order until January 7, 2014. In early January, direct observers of Jahi and at least one physician reported that Jahi regained the ability to self-regulate her core body temperature. Nevertheless, the hospital and court ignored the new evidence of her functioning hypothalamus, a part of her brain that had not irreversibly ceased functioning.

One of the more obvious regulatory functions of the hypothalamus was restored to working order weeks after Jahi was declared dead on December 12, 2013, on the Feast of Our Lady of Guadalupe. Not to digress, but Our Lady of Guadalupe reflects the mission of the Life Guardian Foundation, and we have her image on our website. It was a remarkable occurrence that Jahi's brain death diagnosis was declared on her feast day. On that day, as well, her mother refused to donate Jahi's still-beating heart.

Our Lady of Guadalupe was an apparition of the Virgin Mary, the mother of Jesus, and appeared to Juan Diego in 1531. Juan Diego was the first convert from the Aztecs who practiced human sacrifice by cutting beating hearts out of people. Our Lady of Guadalupe is an appropriate symbol for the Life Guardian Foundation and a spiritual force that opposes the murder of people by cutting out their organs. Our patron Lady is a protector, preserver, and defender of life.

Jahi's misdiagnosis also leads one to wonder how many times other people were preemptively declared dead under the UDDA whole-brain standard according to the AAN guidelines but still had brain function. Such a dynamic, or trend, of extraordinarily and scientifically "restored" brain function, is inconsistent with "irreversible cessation of all functions of the entire brain." It suggests a degree of recovery from brain injury. Jahi's brain was still functioning at a level that could not be detected by expert medical doctors and highly sophisticated diagnostic medical equipment. Yet, she was still declared dead by the whole-brain standard.

CWB: After Jahi was declared dead on December 12, 2013, how was she treated?

PAB: She wasn't treated like a living person but a corpse. The physicians, nurses, and administrators were insensitive, dismissive, and cruel. They flipped the narrative around. Children's Hospital Oakland said to the court that it would be unethical and "grotesque" to require the institution and its healthcare professionals to provide further medical care to a dead body, which meant no tracheostomy or feeding tube.

Jahi's mother was portrayed as ignorant, superstitious, and in denial about her daughter's "death." Jahi was discriminated against. Christopher Dolan was characterized as a lawyer craving the limelight. I was painted as "a crusader with an ideology-based bias," trying to advance my private agenda. Jahi's mother was willing to keep medical support going to preserve her life. According to the hospital, if organ donation was not an option, it was time to withdraw medical support and free up the ICU bed for another person more worthy of ongoing life who, incidentally, can also increase the revenue of Children's Hospital Oakland.

Even though Jahi was treated like a corpse — one with a beating heart (circulation), aerating lungs (respiration), and functioning hypothalamus (brain and body integration) on a ventilator — she had remarkable resiliency. After causing suffocation and brain swelling, not once but three times, by performing three separate apnea tests, denying her nutrition, and restricting neuroprotective medications, she still had a measure of healing. One must wonder how much more she would have recovered if Children's Hospital Oakland did not have a policy of death.

After the heated court battle with the hospital, Jahi was finally transferred to a new facility, and the treatment she needed was implemented. She underwent a tracheostomy, had a feeding tube inserted into her belly, and was administered neuroprotective hormones. Now, her brain was able to rest and heal. Jahi's mother was also treated with dignity and respect. Those who valued her life could focus on providing the loving care Jahi needed.

Jahi was trapped "behind enemy lines" in an institutional warzone with only a slim chance of escape. Children's Hospital Oakland did everything in its power to hide the fact that she was alive and to save face by obfuscating her discharge. Jahi escaped from the institution's life unworthy of life minions and eventually journeyed to an apartment on a portable ventilator with a feeding tube. In this compassionate and loved-filled environment, she experienced healing, recovery, care, and her inalienable rights as a US citizen.

What an awful experience for a twenty-first-century teenager and family in the "land of the free" that once opposed the tyranny of England during the American Revolution and slavery during the Civil War and fought against the Nazis in World War II.

On February 1, 2014, Dr. Byrne published: "Jahi McMath, Can You Move," an article that covers much of what was already written above. However, a brief section will be reproduced with some editing and in collaboration with Dr. Byrne.

A video recording that shows an ice cube placed on the bottom of Jahi's right foot was distributed three weeks after she was declared dead. Her foot moved in response to the application of the frozen block. Someone unseen, perhaps it was Jahi's mother, says: "I don't understand how a 'brain-dead' girl can…" and the video ends. I suspect anyone who watched the video would finish the sentence by saying, "…move her foot."

Only a learned neurologist with the authority to declare a person "brain dead" and, therefore, meriting a death certificate under US law wouldn't finish the sentence that way. A neurologist is legally free to declare "brain death" under many "accepted medical standards," but an ice cube to the foot is not one of them. Perhaps it should be. It worked to illicit Jahi's brain and body response.

The next piece, "For the Love of Jahi, the Living Testimony of Nailah Winkfield," was published by Dr. Byrne with help from a colleague, and it appeared on February 7, 2014. The article chronicles Jahi's experience from the beginning of her ordeal and her mother's pleas to show her teenage girl compassion. It also illustrates Nailah's persistent fight against the dehumanizing Goliaths of America. The essay is reproduced below with editing and in collaboration with Dr. Byrne.

Nailah Winkfield's daughter, then twelve-year-old Jahi McMath, suffered from pediatric sleep apnea. On December 9, 2013, Jahi was admitted to Children's Hospital & Research Center Oakland, where she underwent a tonsillectomy and adenoidectomy. Post-op, Jahi asked for a Popsicle and stated that her throat hurt. Most assuredly, Nailah was relieved, knowing her beloved Jahi was doing well. Then, there was a sudden, dreadful turn of events. Unknown to everyone, Jahi was secretly bleeding, and it was ignored by medical staff until it became a medical emergency. The bleeding complication from the surgery continued until Jahi's heart stopped and her brain lost oxygen.

Nailah was informed of this turn of events after

Jahi was resuscitated and put on a ventilator. She was also told at this time that Jahi had brain damage due to decreased circulation to her brain. The brain damage was said to have progressed, and then on Tuesday, December 10, Nailah was informed that Jahi was "brain dead." On Thursday, December 12, Jahi was declared "medically" and "legally" dead. Nailah refused organ donation from Jahi and thus began her fight for Jahi's life, ironically, after an arduous court battle and her daughter's legal certification of death!

Although on a ventilator, Nailah witnessed her daughter's vital signs on the monitor moving in unison with a rhythmic procession across the screen as Jahi's heart continued to beat. Jahi's heart has pumped blood throughout her body and brain more than three million times since her surgery. The brain is not necessary for the heart to beat. Nailah held Jahi, and she felt the warmth of her daughter—her still living Jahi. Nailah prayed for healing, and while clinging to her faith, the hope of Jahi's recovery remained. On the other hand, Children's Hospital Oakland treated Jahi like a corpse, and Nailah had to fight tooth and nail to protect and preserve her daughter's life.

Even though the doctors and hospital administrators would deny Jahi medically necessary treatments, Nailah would not relent. She was like the woman in Jesus' parable about the unjust judge, who persevered until her request was heard and granted. Nailah continued to fight for Jahi's life, and the judge entered a stay on Jahi's execution. Now, Nailah could transfer Jahi to another facility for medically necessary treatment. However, the doctors, lawyers, and administrators at Children's Hospital Oakland persisted in their murderous efforts to remove Jahi from the ventilator.

They did everything possible to prevent Jahi's transfer to a more compassionate institution. Nailah prevailed with the help of her lawyer, Christopher Dolan.

Many negative comments were written about Nailah and Jahi, but that's the death-dealing "life unworthy of life" culture America has become in the twenty-first century. Murder the mentally disabled because they are a useless financial burden to society and harvest their still-living body parts for those deemed more worthy to live. Many can be excused for their comments simply because they have limited knowledge. Yet some, as they propagate this death-dealing and dehumanizing agenda, seem to be trying to hurt and humiliate Nailah and Jahi.

Nailah is a mother whose love transcends medical terminology, legal technicalities, monetary means, public opinion, and any form of social persuasion. Nailah's commitment to protecting and preserving her daughter's life is admirable, not a delusional denial of reality. She is aware of Jahi's condition; the deluded ones are those who do not recognize a beating heart, respiration, circulation, and a functioning hypothalamus, indicating brain and body integration as ongoing life — not only under the flawed definition of the UDDA but also by the standard of commonsense.

These are the delusional dupes who deny the facts of science and the inalienable rights of all American citizens, including Jahi. They also disregard a mother's love for her daughter. At the very least, everyone, in some way, should be able to relate to that, namely, a mother who did not have an abortion and carried them and brought them into the world.

We are privileged to observe this mother's gallant fight for her daughter's life and her continued love and nurturing amid the adversity of *the defamatory and discriminatory hordes* who do not recognize *their* moment-by-moment dependency on air, food, and other people to survive. You see in Nailah the conviction, resolve, and boldness of Friedrich Bonhoeffer to confront the evil of Nazism, and we witness God's boundless love, mercy, and grace in action for her disabled daughter. Thank you, Nailah!

The following article, "Jahi McMath—Accepting Her Life," published by Dr. Byrne on March 18, 2014, recapitulates much of the material already presented in this book. Its unique contribution shows how these concerns shape and play out in real life. The piece responds to the National Catholic Bioethics Center's (NCBC) commitment to Jahi's brain death diagnosis and how the organization's position is at odds with official Roman Catholic teaching. Again, the essay is reproduced below with editing and after collaboration with Dr. Byrne.

Dead is dead—except when it isn't. The National Catholic Bioethics Center (NCBC) ethicists have repeatedly claimed that Jahi McMath is dead. Yet, Jahi continues to live. Jahi is Jahi, not a dead body receiving treatment, care, and love. Jahi may be called a corpse, but she is not a corpse; she is a living human being.

Before the desire to get beating hearts and other healthy vital organs for transplantation, physicians cautiously determined death in order not to treat the living as dead. Then, illegal and immoral heart transplantation began. To make it legal, in 1968, a committee at Harvard concocted the first set of "brain death" criteria (not based on scientific investigation) known as the Harvard Criteria. During the next ten years, thirty disparate sets of criteria were published, each one tending to be less stringent. In a 2010 edition of *Neurology*, the publishers admitted there was a lack of consensus about which criteria to use when determining brain death, and the brain-related criteria used were not based on scientific evidence.

The NCBC ethicists refer to an address by Pope John Paul II to support their position on brain death as death. The pontiff stated the "criterion ...does not seem to conflict with essential elements of sound anthropology." The use of "seem" *seems* to indicate that there are some unanswered questions. It *seems* the "criterion" for brain death must not "conflict with essential elements of sound anthropology." To understand what he means by the word "seem" would require a face-to-face inquiry, but since the pope is dead, we cannot do this. The best we can do today is evaluate his other writings.

Pope John Paul II later wrote: "Each human being, in fact, is alive precisely insofar as he or she is *corpore et anima unus*, and he or she remains so for as long as this substantial unity-in-totality subsists. In the light of this anthropological truth, it is clear, as I have already had occasion to observe, that 'the death of the person, understood in this primary sense, is an event which no scientific technique or empirical method can identify directly.'" Science cannot determine the moment the *anima* or life force or spirit or soul separates from the body, and there is nothing in this statement about the brain being the animating principle of life. It *seems* the Pope is ruling out brain death as a definition of death altogether when other signs of life are present. Thus, the *anima* has not separated from the body.

Does the declaration of death under the legal "accepted medical standards" make Jahi genuinely dead? The NCBC ethicists have access to court records indicating that Jahi's heart is still beating, and she has normal blood pressure, temperature, and respiration but requires a ventilator. The ventilator pushes air into Jahi. The living Jahi pushes the air out. Does every NCBC ethicist agree that Jahi is no longer "*corpore et unus*"? If they say that Jahi's *anima*, life, spirit, or soul is not in "*unus*" — united with her body — then what is ultimately behind her beating heart, aerating lungs, and other bodily functions?

The emphasis by neurologists and NCBC ethicists is on removing the ventilator that supports the need for Jahi's inspiratory act of breathing. In declaring "brain death," turning off the ventilator becomes a question only after organ donation is refused. If Jahi's mother answered yes to organ harvesting, then Jahi's organs would have been dissected out — this would have ended her life, not the withdrawal of the ventilator. Jahi's heart would be beating in someone else. Yes, Jahi would die after her beating heart and other vital organs had been removed, and the ventilator would not be withdrawn.

The NCBC ethicists note that "an independent court-appointed pediatric neurologist from Stanford University" found nothing different from the original conclusions by the doctors at Children's Hospital Oakland. Did anyone expect a court-appointed neurologist to see something different? The NCBC ethicists also note, "The coroner's office has issued a death certificate." Yes, a death certificate was required for Jahi's mother to get her daughter out of the clutches of those determined to end Jahi's life! The Bureau of Vital Statistics recorded Jahi's death. It was the first time a death certificate was issued for someone with a beating heart and respiration. When a non-donor is declared "brain dead," a death certificate is typically not given until there are no signs of life.

Two essential doctrines underlie the Roman Catholic understanding of life and death: (1) The soul is the principle of life or *anima*. Death is the separation of the soul from the body. A spiritual essence exists where it operates. We know the soul is still present because we see its operations in the body of Jahi. Therefore, Jahi is not dead and does not meet the condition laid down by Pope John Paul II on August 29, 2000, for harvesting organs: "Vital organs which occur singly in the body can be removed only after death, that is, from the body of someone who is certainly dead." Pope Benedict XVI reiterated this on November 7, 2008: "Individual vital organs cannot be extracted except *ex cadavere*," or until the person is a non-heart-beating corpse. (2) When in doubt, we must presume in favor life, yes, Jahi's life, to protect the dignity and sanctity of the person as a human being created in the image and likeness of God—life and being are gifts from the Creator of life and must be cherished and defended.

"Brain death" is one of the leading causes of the dehumanization of people in our culture today. We are treating the living as dead for utilitarian purposes—namely, to harvest organs for financial gain and to provide ongoing life for those deemed more worthy of living than the mentally disabled who still have signs of life. We are looking at fellow image-bearers of the Creator of life as NAPA body-part stores! The view of the NCBC has never been in the mind of the Roman Catholic Church, nor is the organization's position in accord with Pope John Paul II's thoughts and wishes as expressed in *The Gospel of Life*.

The faithful in the Church will not endorse the ending of Jahi's life. Unfortunately, the NCBC is misguided about its affirmation of brain death as death, and the organization needs to repent and stop leading Christians astray. Jahi is alive, and she is living. She is a precious child created in the image and likeness of God, even though she is on a ventilator and requires a feeding tube. The church is called upon to pray for Jahi and all those caring for her and ignore the life-dishonoring, immoral, and unethical guidance offered by the NCBC.

In October 2014, attorney Christopher Dolan filed a motion with the California Superior Court requesting a reversal of Jahi's legal status of death. According to California law, she was not entitled to financial assistance for ongoing care since she was legally dead. Dr. Shewmon provided testimony on Jahi's behalf. He declared to the court: "I can assert unequivocally that Jahi currently does not fulfill diagnostic criteria for brain death." Further, Dr. Shewmon stated: "She is an extremely disabled but very much alive teenage girl."

Not surprisingly, but sadly, the California court upheld Jahi's death certificate. However, that judgment would be revisited. On May 21, 2015, a jubilant Dr. Byrne published "Jahi is Alive—Praise the Lord and Pass the Ammunition," which chronicled his visit to see Jahi in New Jersey, along with some reflections on issues relating to life and death. A summary of the encounter is recorded below with editing, minus the thoughts already covered in this chapter.

Recently, I visited Jahi and her family at her home in New Jersey. Jahi's heart has continued to beat more than sixty million times since she was declared 'brain dead.' The Children's Hospital Oakland doctors told Nailah that her heart would stop beating or that she would start the decomposition process if the ventilator were not withdrawn. Neither has happened. It's nearly two years later, and these predictions have not occurred. Jahi has been alive since conception inside her mother, and Jahi is alive with a brain injury fourteen years later and is showing signs of improvement.

The day I visited was beautiful. It wasn't just a lovely sunny day with a clear blue sky, but a day filled with the sunshine of Jahi and her loving mother by her side. There she was, lying relaxed with a bright, shiny-black complexion. What a beautiful girl! One who bears the image and likeness of the Creator of life. Like most teenagers, Jahi was wearing lip gloss. I held hands with Jahi, and Nailah took a picture of our clasped hands. That picture and the rubber wristbands we share are precious to me. The one on the right wrist says, 'Prayer Works,' and on the left, 'Jahi Lives.'

On September 21, 2017, Dr. Byrne published "Judge Rules Jahi McMath May NOT Be Dead." In this article, Dr. Byrne reflects on Jahi's case since her diagnosis of brain death and presents how the lack of treatment at Children's Hospital Oakland influenced her prognosis. He also mentions the institution's violation of the ethical principles of non-maleficence and beneficence. His essay is reproduced below, after collaboration with Dr. Byrne and editing.

Jahi McMath is alive in New Jersey! Four years after she was declared dead in California, a judge in California has ruled that Jahi may not be dead after all. Jahi's lawyer, Christopher Dolan, explains the turn of events:
> Legal proceedings in both the state and federal courts were ongoing throughout this time to prove Jahi was alive. In a medical negligence case, judges repeatedly ruled that the facts created a triable issue of fact that Jahi was alive.

As the brain-death statute required that there needed to be total and irreversible cessation of all neurological activity, the judges ruled that there was evidence which should be presented to a jury for them to decide if Jahi was alive or not.

There is evidence that the whole-brain death statute under the UDDA was not met since Jahi has exhibited brain function, which indicates medical negligence due to misdiagnosis. Dolan provides some background events that led to the judge's ruling.

> Over those four years, Jahi began communicating in response to her mother's voice. She could move her fingers, hands and feet in response to requests by her mother and eventually could signal yes or no. ...peer-reviewed articles were published by experts, including Dr. Calixto Machado, a neurologist seen as one of the premier international brain-death experts, which showed that electroencephalographic testing (EEG) showed that Jahi had brain-wave activity, and MRIs of the brain showed that it was, while severely damaged, still intact. In a case of total brain death, the brain liquifies and is absorbed into the body. This did not happen in Jahi's case.

Neither the California statute nor the practice of medicine ought to be significantly different in any other state in recognizing the essential difference between a living person with a beating heart and circulation, albeit on a ventilator, versus the remains of a dead body. Jahi is a case in point, but unfortunately, she was treated as if she were a corpse when she was not.

What is the problem? There is no problem in New Jersey because, although alone among the fifty states, New Jersey law rightly recognizes that a person cannot be declared "brain dead" if the person in a written document or the family objects to this view of "death," and embraces the time-honored universally recognized irreversible cessation of circulation and respiration as determining death.

However, there are problems in the remaining forty-nine states. For example, Nevada has made "brain death" criteria an absolute standard of death without recourse to challenge it. Doctors can declare a person's brain dead and, therefore, dead in Nevada. If you want to give a "brain dead" loved one with a beating heart on a ventilator time to heal or to be transferred to a nursing care facility or a home on a portable ventilator, those requests will be denied. After declaring brain death, unless the person is an organ donor, medications will be stopped, tubes pulled, and medical devices turned off.

A request to continue ventilator support seems reasonable considering the controversy surrounding brain death as death, and the courts in California recognized it as such, but this is not the case in Nevada. With the new "brain death" law in Nevada, Jahi would not have made it to New Jersey. Life-sustaining treatment will be withdrawn when the doctor declares "brain death." If a medical proxy objects, expensive medical bills for ongoing "organ-sustaining" treatment must be paid out of pocket. The person is "dead" in Nevada, so private insurance, Medicare, and Medicaid reimbursement end, and if out-of-pocket payment cannot be made, treatment stops.

Thankfully, the Superior Court in California

stopped further actions that would have ended Jahi's life. Without Jahi's mother and her attorney fighting for judicial intervention, Jahi's ventilator would have been turned off. Jahi would be dead and buried, which is what Children's Hospital Oakland wanted. The uncomfortable truth about the deception of "brain death" would still be safely tucked away and hidden from the public eye.

Questions like, how can a dead person have a beating heart? Regulate body temperature and blood pressure? Excrete waste products? Metabolize nutrition? Heal wounds? Move a foot in response to coolness? Go through puberty? Experience menses? Eventually, move on command? Demonstrate neurological healing using some of the same tests that were used to declare her dead! These questions, and many more, would have never crossed people's minds. The fact is "brain death" is a lie. If anything is "fake" in modern times, it is "brain death."

It is essential to understand that Jahi was never truly dead in California. If Jahi had been treated like a living person with a brain injury rather than a brain-dead corpse, her chances of healing and recovery would have dramatically improved. She was denied medically necessary treatment at Oakland Children's Hospital, and the hospital did not provide nutrition for thirty days. After being transported to New Jersey, Jahi was administered thyroid hormone, received a tracheostomy, and had proper nutrition via a feeding tube.

The Children's Hospital Oakland denied Jahi routine treatments with potential benefits and performed the harmful apnea test three times! The apnea test is an "acid test" for "brain death" that causes suffocation for up to ten minutes because the inspiratory aspect of breathing is stopped when the ventilator is turned off. Carbon dioxide, an acid waste product that can harm the body in large doses, increases to levels that supposedly will result in the person attempting to breathe. If the person can't, or carbon dioxide goes above certain levels in the blood, he or she is declared "brain dead." The apnea test does nothing to benefit the brain-injured person but only causes harm.

The main point is that even though Jahi couldn't breathe then and may still not be able to do so now, she was and is alive with a beating heart, circulation, respiration, and brain and body integration. The issue has implications for Jahi's right to life and many others who have lost consciousness and do not take a breath when a ventilator is removed. After Jahi's mother did not grant permission to take Jahi's organs, Children's Hospital Oakland wanted to stop the ventilator and kill her to free up the bed for a patient deemed more worthy of ongoing care. In hospitals across America, this is now standard practice.

The determination of death based on neurological criteria, or the whole-brain formulation of death, requires the demonstration of "irreversible cessation of all functions of the entire brain, including the brain stem." In practice, this is believed to occur when all the brain's blood vessels (arteries, capillaries, and veins) are fully or nearly fully compressed by intracranial pressure (ICP). Increased ICP is usually the result of brain swelling that occurs after the acute phase of brain damage due to head trauma, an infection, bleeding, or the loss of oxygen.

Expansion of brain edema or swelling is caused by the accumulation of excess fluids, similar to swelling that occurs after a sprained ankle. In other words, ICP increases when the brain volume expands within the inelastic cranial vault or skull. In Jahi, increased ICP was associated with a lack of oxygen due to the loss of blood in the brain (the trauma), repeated apnea tests, and the increase of fluid to cause swelling in response to those injuries.

Often, blood flow studies are never performed on people declared dead under the UDDA neurological standard. Due to the controversy surrounding Jahi, blood flow imaging studies were conducted. Jahi met those additional diagnostic criteria for the UDDA neurological standard in December 2013. She was declared "brain dead" by three physicians at Children's Hospital Oakland and ultimately by the chief of pediatric neurology at Stanford University School of Medicine, appointed by the court to act as an independent examiner. The accepted diagnostic criteria for "brain death" went above and beyond the commonly applied "accepted medical standards." These doctors meticulously applied, verified, and recorded the results of their testing. Nevertheless, Jahi was still misdiagnosed, so treatment was not administered to help her heal and recover.

The court-appointed expert testified that the brain blood flow study revealed "no cerebral blood flow." Yet, recent blood flow studies demonstrate that much of Jahi's brain structure is preserved, which means she never lost blood flow. She had a condition called "global ischemic penumbra," which is common in victims of cardiovascular accidents or strokes. Although Jahi's case was severe, the goal of treatment for this condition is to reverse oxygen deprivation, not increase it by apnea tests, and to rush to a declaration of death.

Jahi never experienced "irreversible cessation of all functions of the entire brain, including the brain stem." Not to mention, a part of her brain called the hypothalamus regulated her core body temperature, and later, Jahi experienced menses, both of which require brain and body integration. Then, of course, Jahi started to move on command. Now, Jahi is not even in a coma but has conscious awareness.

What immediate treatment would have helped reverse the "global ischemic penumbra" Jahi experienced? The administration of thyroid hormone. Hormone production by the thyroid gland can only occur under brain stimulation and the hypothalamus. The administration of thyroid hormone supplements to the thyroid gland increases thyroid hormone production and reduces inflammation in the brain.

When someone experiences a head injury, brain edema progresses, brain circulation is restricted due to an increase in ICP, and the thyroid gland reduces the production of thyroid hormones. Not enough thyroid hormone worsens brain edema (a medical condition called myxedema). A vicious cycle is set into motion, where brain edema causes reduced thyroid hormone synthesis, which, in turn, worsens brain edema. In other words, a severely sick brain leads to an unhealthy thyroid gland and to a worsening of a person's brain injury. At some point, the person is in a state of "global ischemic penumbra," which is mistakenly diagnosed as "brain death" and leads to the destruction of neurological tissue if it is untreated.

Children's Hospital Oakland violated two principles of medical ethics: non-maleficence and beneficence. The second principle requires medical professionals to attempt to achieve maximum therapeutic benefit for their patients. Although the importance of thyroid hormones for the brain has been a part of solid medical knowledge for decades, Children's Hospital Oakland refused to administer it to Jahi. Administering the hormone would have helped achieve maximum therapeutic benefit for Jahi. Adequate nutrition would have been beneficial as well. The second principle, nonmaleficence, means "above all, do no harm" to your patient. Jahi was harmed by apnea tests, lack of adequate treatment, and the cold attitude of healthcare providers who viewed her as a corpse.

Jahi is alive and has always been alive. If she were cared for as if she were alive, her chances of recovery would have dramatically improved, and her care would have been ethical.

As Jahi's case to vacate her false death sentence was being prepared, she died on June 22, 2018. Liver failure, which led to a cardiac arrest while on the ventilator, was her cause of death. Now, the legal debate is over which death certificate is valid! Her lawyer explains:

The California Death Certificate was never completed or signed, as required by law, by any attending physician. The New Jersey Death Certificate is full, complete and final, being duly executed after an autopsy.

Why was the death certificate in California

incomplete? Jahi didn't experience cardiopulmonary cessation, and no doctor would declare someone *de facto* dead with a beating heart!

The effect of Jahi's ongoing life for nearly five years raised renewed awareness about brain death as a legitimate definition of death. On April 11, 2018, Harvard Medical School hosted: "Defining Death: Organ Transplantation and the 50-Year Legacy of the Harvard Report on Brain Death." Experts on both sides presented their views about the legitimacy of brain death, and several presentations included references to Jahi. The prevailing consensus among the experts was that the UDDA is a legal fiction. Then, on November 3, 2021, under pressure from the American Academy of Neurology (AAN), the Uniform Law Commission (ULC) reconvened to attempt a revision of the seriously flawed UDDA.

Dependent Jahi on a ventilator with a feeding tube exposed the fallacy of brain death. Jahi and many others, Aden Hailu, Charlie Gard, Israel Stinson, Alan Callaway, and Areen Chakrabarti, inspired Dr. Byrne to continue his tireless fight to protect and defend the lives of vulnerable people with renewed vigor. With the door open for revisions to the UDDA with the ULC, Dr. Byrne saw the opportunity to take the bold step of attempting to repeal and replace the UDDA.

4

"The Uniform Determination of Death Act (UDDA): Repeal and Replace"

According to a January 27, 2023 "Brain Death Criteria" education activity that provides standard protocol instructions for healthcare providers published by *StatPearls*: "Brain death accounts for around 2% of deaths in the United States and is often caused by traumatic brain injury."

In 2022, approximately 3,273,705 deaths occurred in the United States (US), which means roughly 65,474 people were declared dead based on death by neurological criteria (DNC). The activity also states: "Criteria for brain death determination were published in the American Academy of Neurology [AAN] guidelines, *but they are still a topic of ongoing debate*" (emphasis mine).

Two percent sounds insignificant, but in context to the number of deaths in 2022, those 65,474 people declared dead by DNC would fill to maximum capacity most National Football League (NFL) stadiums.

In clinical practice, the diagnosis of brain death includes a lot of technical jargon and expert opinions, and it is often made during an emotionally charged crisis. Much depends on interpreting this specialized information from medical authorities for whom the *debate is settled* — "brain death" equals the death of a person. As noted numerous times throughout this book, the ideological framework supporting brain death as death is rooted in utilitarianism, not the biological sciences, and it discriminates against the mentally disabled.

The AAN clumps all types of "brain death" together, even if a person does not have an obliterated brain or decapitated head, which is vital for the public to know. The AAN has determined that a non-responsive person with a still-beating heart, circulation, respiration, and a level of neurological activity on a ventilator will be considered dead when: "Abrupt loss of cerebral perfusion occurs if a concomitant elevation of intracranial pressure is more than mean arterial pressure (cerebral perfusion pressure (CPP) = mean arterial pressure (MAP) - intracranial pressure (ICP)." In lay terms, this means the brain has *supposedly* swelled to the point of preventing blood flow from the heart to maintain *measurable* circulation to the brain.

Jahi McMath met this formula, and then she didn't. According to the educational activity cited already, she had the following type of DNC:

> [B]rain injury, as seen in patients following cardiopulmonary arrest with delayed resuscitation, resulting in prolonged cessation of cerebral blood flow. The resultant anoxia leads to neuronal damage, resulting in cellular membrane pump failure, disturbed osmoregulation, and, ultimately, severe brain edema. As a result of the confined space of the skull, ICP increases, compromising cerebral perfusion and resulting in further neuronal injury.

Several experts interpreting this data diagnosed Jahi with a "prolonged cessation of cerebral blood flow" to the brain. Nevertheless, after extraordinary resilience—Jahi was subjected to three apnea tests, starvation, and being treated like a corpse—with adequate hormonal treatment and time, Jahi experienced reduced brain swelling, increased cerebral perfusion, and measurable neurological healing.

The learned elites following the AAN guidance and interpreting the medical data were proven wrong by Jahi. Perhaps many in the sell-out crowd at the NFL stadium, with time and appropriate care, would have also demonstrated their awful misdiagnosis and exposed their life unworthy of life propaganda. However, no one will ever know what the actual figures of misdiagnosis are because those diagnosed as brain dead by the AAN criteria are murdered by the removal of a ventilator or by having their organs cut out.

There are about 1.7 million organ donors, a 200,000-person increase since 2021. *Registered* organ donors dying in the 2022 pool of 65,474 are *mandated* under the Uniform Anatomical Gift Act (UAGA) to donate their body parts after a declaration of death under the neurological standard of the UDDA. Dr. Byrne mentioned these obligations in an earlier chapter.

People applying for a driver's license have seen the cheery cartoon posters at the Department of Motor Vehicles (DMV) to "Give the Gift of Life." Before signing up, however, to give their own *irreplaceable life* to strangers *deemed more worthy of life*, they are never *informed* about the risks of being an organ donor or this ongoing brain-death controversy. Nor are they made aware that people have recovered from a diagnosis of brain death. Dr. Shewmon suggested a Surgeon General's warning on these DMV posters: "Warning: It remains controversial whether you will actually be dead at the time of the removal of your organs."

As mentioned in the last chapter, on November 3, 2021, the Uniform Law Commission (ULC) reconvened to revise the UDDA due to pressure from the AAN. Physicians across the United States (US) were not following the UDDA's whole-brain definition of death. As a result, they were violating the Dead Donor Rule (DDR) for organ donors and people declared dead under the UDDA. Lawyers were filing lawsuits as a result, and physicians and medical institutions were being sued.

Dr. Byrne saw an opportunity to confront the UDDA head-on and mounted an aggressive attack to protect and defend life. On *Renew America*, seven months before the first meeting (March 15, 2021), he published "The Uniform Determination of Death Act (UDDA): Repeal and Replace." The article is reproduced below with collaboration from Dr. Byrne and after editing.

The Uniform Determination of Death Act (UDDA) has been adopted in all fifty states based on the recommendations of the Uniform Law Commission (ULC). However, not all the states in the country use identical language. Now, the ULC is considering revising the UDDA.

Revising the UDDA is a good idea, but only if the revision will correct the problems with the current UDDA by replacing it with a model statute that protects life until the end of biological life, not "brain death." A person's death is the cessation of physical life on the earth. The precise moment when a person's life ends is paramount since the right to live is inalienable. Under the United States Constitution, the government must protect an American citizen's right to "life, liberty, and the pursuit of happiness."

The UDDA states: "An individual who has sustained either 1) irreversible cessation of circulatory and respiratory functions, or 2) irreversible cessation of all functions of the entire brain, including the brain stem, is dead. A determination of death must be made in accordance with accepted medical standards."

The first (1) "irreversible cessation of circulatory and respiratory functions" has been accepted for eons. "Irreversible" was added by the UDDA, but that had traditionally been determined by waiting sufficient time for destruction to occur so that there would be certainty of a person's death.

The second (2) "irreversible cessation of all functions of the entire brain, including the brain stem," also known as "brain death" or death by neurological criteria (DNC), has always been controversial, even though it is widely practiced in medicine and legally protected under the law.

Ideal statute wording
An ideal statute should be worded in the negative to defend lives. The legal statute should protect the person from being declared dead when he or she might still be alive. Suggested wording in the negative would be: "**No one shall be declared dead unless respiratory and circulatory systems and the entire brain have been destroyed. Such destruction shall be determined in accord with universally accepted medical standards**," which will be described below. "Destruction" of all the body's vital systems supports death as a fact of science, and the negative all-inclusive "no one" safeguards everyone's right to life under the Constitution.

In recent legal cases, loved ones of patients with a beating heart, circulation, and other signs of life had to fight to continue care. These people did not experience the destruction of the three central, vital systems: respiratory, circulatory, and neurological (at least the entire brain). Often, these cases are prosecuted because the medical institutions treating them see their care as futile, but profits drive their concerns. In the 2020 Milliman Report, forty billion was allocated for organ transplants, with six billion by physicians.

The loved ones of Jahi McMath, Israel Stinson, Aden Hailu, Bobby Reyes, Allen Callaway, Miranda Lawson, Areen Chakrabarti, and many others should not have to fight to continue their lives because greedy hospitals want to turn a profit.

In reality, providing care for one "brain-dead" person to get him or her out of an ICU or to die on a ventilator in an ICU is a lot cheaper than the costs to Medicare, Medicaid, and private insurers that medical institutions benefit from, particularly when they harvest body parts from one "brain dead" person and transplant them into numerous people deemed more worthy to live.

Irreversibility

Irreversibility is not an empirical concept—it is not directly observable or provable by experience or experiment. As noted in my 1979 "Brain Death—An Opposing Viewpoint" *JAMA* article:

> Both destruction of the brain and the cessation of its functions are, in principle, directly observable, such observations can serve as evidence. Irreversibility, however, of any kind, is a property about which we can learn only by inference from prior experience. It is not an observable condition. Hence, it cannot serve as evidence, nor can it rightly be made part of an empirical criterion of death. ...if there is no proof of complete destruction, then any declaration that a cessation of function is absolutely irreversible is a presumption, even if well grounded, which is contingent on the current state of medical knowledge and on the availability of adequate life-support systems in the

> concrete circumstances. Even if the presumption is correct, it establishes …no necessary link with destruction of the brain. If it is incorrect, the patient may possibly be cured. Thus, whether right or wrong, a presumption as to the irreversibility of a lack of brain function is insufficient ground for removing a patient's vital organs or for immediate autopsy, cremation, or burial.

Destruction confirms a state of irreversibility, not vice versa.

Importance of "destruction" of circulatory and respiratory systems and the entire brain

It is important to note that "destruction" is the only acceptable interpretation of the phrase "irreversible cessation of all functions." Destruction indicates the loss of structural potentiality for functioning—the cessation of the organic capacity to act.

The diagnosis, condition, or state known as death cannot be reversed by medical treatment. Prognosis, whether of recovery or destruction, is irrelevant to any determination of death, nor is the impossibility of even minimal recovery the same thing as death. Death is death, period—the change from one state of being to another.

Importance of accurate language

Medical personnel may use language about death that is imprecise. For example, doctors may say a person who had a cardiac arrest and was successfully resuscitated had "died" and was brought back to life. However, the doctor's statement is incorrect, and the physician's medical training contradicts this assertion.

The person may have been near death and might have died if an intervention had not been attempted, but he or she was never dead.

Signs of life before and after the declaration of DNC
The public has not been informed that a person declared dead by neurological criteria (DNC) still has a heart beating, circulation, and respiration (exchange of oxygen and carbon dioxide in the tissues albeit on a ventilator). Other signs of life continue, such as wound healing, a complex, diffuse process throughout the body. There is urine production, maintenance of body temperature, homeostasis of many interdependently functioning organs and systems, and, if a woman is pregnant, even the ability to carry and nourish the baby in the womb. Not to mention, several people have recovered and gone on to live regular lives after being diagnosed neurologically dead.

Doctors may refer to the patient declared dead using DNC as a corpse. However, the patient still has signs of life, unlike a genuine corpse, and may even experience a limited or full recovery over time with proper treatment.

Function, functions, functioning
The UDDA states that "all functions of the entire brain" must have ceased for a declaration of death. The brain has many functions, some continuing even after "brain death" is declared. To exclude some functions, but not all, does not meet the statutory requirement of "irreversible cessation of *all functions* of the *entire brain*, including the *brainstem*" (emphasis mine).

The Supreme Court in Nevada unanimously (7-0) ruled that the case of Aden Hailu be sent back to the lower court because they were not convinced that the hospital's use of the American Academy of Neurology (AAN) guidelines fulfilled the statutory requirement of "irreversible cessation of all functions of the entire brain including the brain stem." Although widely used, the AAN criteria are not evidence-based and do not fulfill the statutory requirement of the UDDA. Nevertheless, Nevada now follows the AAN standards. Without input from voters, state legislators in Nevada changed the law. Now, a determination of death by the model UDDA neurological standard must be made according to the AAN guidelines.

Neurologist Dr. Alan Shewmon states: "It has long been recognized that in some cases of clinically diagnosed brain death, certain brain structures may not only be preserved but actually function, such as the hypothalamus." In clinical practice, this is always true of "brain dead" people without diabetes insipidus, low thyroid hormone, or the inability to maintain temperature control. Absence of functioning does not necessarily mean cessation of all functions in people declared dead under the AAN-inspired DNC criteria. Still, the AAN permits these functions to be present while a person is considered a corpse.

The UDDA has sought to turn a "cessation of all brain functions of the entire brain, including the brainstem," into a general criterion to define death. As noted in the same article cited above, "to take *that which functions* to be simply identical with its *functioning*" is to make "a fundamental category mistake." Further, "if something irreversibly ceases to function, its existence is not necessarily extinguished; it merely becomes *permanently* idle. Nonfunction, no matter what prognostic qualifiers are used with it, is not the same thing as destruction." For example, when an automobile is parked, it is not functioning, but the functions are still there to make the car move. After the automobile is broken beyond repair, it is no longer idle, and it ceases to be an automobile but is an amalgamation of metal that cannot function.

Accepted medical standards
Many sets of criteria for declaring death by DNC have been considered "accepted medical standards," beginning with the Harvard Criteria in 1968. Between 1968 and 1978, more than thirty sets of different criteria were considered "accepted medical standards." The AAN proposes a revised Uniform Determination of Death Act (rUDDA), effectively making the AAN guidelines and any future updates the only "accepted" medical standard. This standard is now codified as law in Nevada.

The AAN standards do not evaluate all brain functions
Unless all functions of the entire brain are evaluated, it is impossible to determine that all functions have ceased. Laboratory tests show that parts of the brain, such as the hypothalamus, may still function and secrete hormones needed for the body. If a loved one has a brain injury and "brain death" is being considered, it is reasonable to demand that blood tests for thyroid stimulating hormone (TSH), T3, T4, and other hormones such as adrenocorticotropic hormone (ACTH) be performed. The AAN standards require ruling out endocrine abnormalities before diagnosing brain death. No revisions of the UDDA should allow patients with parts of the brain still functioning to be declared dead.

The procedure of the apnea test
One function of the brainstem part of the brain is to take a breath. When carbon dioxide increases in the blood, it stimulates receptors in the brainstem, which, in turn, causes the inspiratory action for breathing. When the brain swells and circulation is impaired, the brainstem is pressed down into the body, and the ability to breathe is impaired. A procedure called the apnea test is often performed to evaluate the spontaneous inspiratory breathing function of the brainstem.

The person must be on a ventilator to be considered for DNC. The apnea test is performed after the unconscious brain-injured person does not respond to noxious stimuli or voice commands and does not show the functioning of *some* brainstem reflexes. It's important to note that all the brainstem reflexes are not tested, and this factor alone negates the "irreversible cessation of all functions of the entire brain, including the brainstem." Thus, the apnea test could be used as a shortcut to declare death by the UDDA respiratory standard since it evaluates the inspiratory function of the brainstem.

The apnea test includes a complete disconnection of the person from the ventilator, sometimes leaving him or her unable to breathe for up to ten minutes. The inability to inspire air causes the waste products of carbon dioxide and acids to increase. If the patient is not observed to breathe or gasp during this time and the arterial blood gas sample shows a carbon dioxide level of at least 60 mmHg or 20 mmHg above baseline, the patient may be declared officially dead.

Often, physicians, without notice or consent, perform the apnea test because they consider it part of their "neurological exam." However, it is more appropriately termed a "procedure" because the life-preserving ventilator is removed, and oxygen may be administered. The procedure has other steps, such as obtaining arterial blood samples. Complete information should be provided to the family. The apnea test has the risk of causing further brain injury and even death.

The apnea test has no clinical benefit for the brain-injured person. Adverse changes in blood pressure and increased carbon dioxide can worsen brain swelling. Other side effects reported during the apnea test are low oxygen (hypoxemia), arrhythmias, pneumothorax, subcutaneous emphysema, pulmonary hypertension, heart attack, and death.

The people who may meet the criteria for the apnea test are already critically ill and unstable. Brief episodes of low blood pressure may adversely harm the already injured brain. Usually, deliberate increases in carbon dioxide are contraindicated in the care of brain-injured patients. Even if oxygen is administered during the apnea test, this does not prevent the potentially lethal effects of increased carbon dioxide on brain swelling. In addition, giving oxygen may depress the reflex to breathe since it may only be low oxygen to which some brainstem centers would respond.

The apnea test has no value for the critically ill and unstable brain-injured person, and it violates the ethical principles of beneficence and nonmaleficence.

Reasons to repeal and replace UDDA
Death is the absence of life on the earth. The US Constitution protects an American citizen's right to life. There should be only one universally accepted

medical standard for determining death since only one irreversible change occurs when a living person becomes a corpse. After actual death, whatever happens to the remains of the body, whether it involves putrefaction, embalming, or cremation, is describable in terms of destruction, disintegration, and dissolution of the formerly present human being. No one should be declared dead unless life has ceased and death has genuinely occurred.

What can you do? Please write to the Uniform Law Commission (ULC) and tell them that the UDDA needs to be repealed and replaced by (1) **No one shall be declared dead unless respiratory and circulatory systems and the entire brain have been destroyed. Such destruction shall be determined in accord with universally accepted medical standards.** (2) Complete information about testing and the opportunity to decline harmful procedures be provided before death is declared by neurological criteria or DNC.

After Dr. Byrne published "The Uniform Determination of Death Act (UDDA): Repeal and Replace" on March 15, 2021, he produced a form letter for the ULC on June 19, 2023, with mailing instructions, along with help from his colleague Dr. Christine Zainer, an anesthesiologist. Below is Dr. Byrne's plea to the *Renew America* audience.

Dear Friends of Life,
Medical and legal elites want the Uniform Law Commission (ULC) to change the Uniform Determination

of Death Act (UDDA) to make "brain death" easier to declare, explicitly without consent, including for the apnea test which removes the life-supporting ventilator and only risks harm.

Conscience opt-outs have been discussed, but only if objection is made "prior" to initiating the "brain death" exam protocol. Physician and healthcare provider opt-outs were not included. Conscience rights must include both patients and providers.

Before presenting the form letter prepared by Drs. Byrne and Zainer, it will be helpful to consider the reasons for reconvening the ULC and the requested changes. The UDDA was passed into law in 1981. Much debate has occurred as to whether the standards bypass the Dead Donor Rule (DDR), which states that removing organs from donors cannot be the cause of death for these people.

When organs are harvested from people declared brain dead, they still have a beating heart. In donation after circulatory death, these people still have activity in the brain. From a biological standpoint, organ donors declared dead under the UDDA are alive when removing their organs, so they don't meet the DDR.

It is also now a well-established fact that the

whole-brain standard, as proposed by the UDDA, has never actually occurred in anyone declared dead. Hypothalamic function often continues, not all brainstem reflexes are tested, and neurological activity is still present. The AAN proposed a revision to the UDDA (rUDDA) to loosen the requirements and standardize testing in all fifty states that reflect the present policies in Nevada. The ULC is considering these revisions.

The first change would replace the term "irreversible" with "permanent," which means no attempt will be made to reverse the situation, not that the problem cannot be changed. The subsequent alteration would narrow the definition of brain death from "the entire brain," referred to as the "whole-brain formulation," to selected brainstem functions. Another modification aims to standardize DNC testing across medical institutions in the US. Since "accepted medical standards" aren't defined by the UDDA. The final change concerns eliminating the need to obtain informed consent before any neurological exam, including the apnea test, to determine death.

With this background in mind, Drs. Byrne and Zainer drafted the following form letter:

In light of the fact that you [ULC] may be revising the Uniform Determination of Death Act (UDDA), this urgent letter strongly encourages you to *repeal* and *replace* the current UDDA with the model statute below.

The new Act must protect life until death (certain death, no evidence of biological life). Death is the cessation of the person's life on earth. The soul or life force, not any one body part, is the unifying life principle. The precise moment when the soul, the immaterial life force, separates from the body is of paramount importance. Nevertheless, the precise moment for this invisible event is unknowable, and only after the visible event of irreversible cessation of heart and lung function can it be known.

There is no ground for legal presumption or less secure criteria. The right to live is the most basic right. The State is obligated to protect the person's right to live until death. This obligation is independent of any other interest, assuming innocence of a capital crime.

The public has not been informed that a person declared dead by neurological criteria (DNC), i.e., "brain death" (BD) has a beating heart, circulation, and respiration (exchange of oxygen and carbon dioxide) albeit with a ventilator. Urine production, digestion, waste excretion, wound healing, temperature maintenance, and homeostasis of interdependently functioning organs and systems are present. There is the ability to carry and nourish the baby in the womb if pregnant. The BD patient may be called a "corpse," but is not a corpse and is not suitable for burial, cremation, or vital, unpaired organ excision. BD criteria are based on bedside observation of lack of functions, presumed to be "irreversible" or "permanent," neither of which can be tested empirically. They do not require necrosis or destruction. The apnea test is part of BD testing. During the apnea test procedure, the life-supporting ventilator is disconnected for up to 10 minutes. There are no benefits to the patient, only risks of harm.

1. The statute ought to protect the person from being declared dead when still alive. Full and complete information about the apnea test and any tests used to declare BD must be provided with freedom, at any time, by patients, surrogates, physicians, and other health care providers to decline or cease the apnea test, exams, and protocols, for the determination and declaration of BD.

2. Treatment options ought to be made available that protect and preserve the life of the patient, even if disability is a potential outcome. Treatments should not be denied based on "quality-of-life" judgments by caregivers even though a patient or surrogate may legitimately refuse them.

3. The model statute below, in the negative, sets minimum criteria before death is declared. This minimum fulfills a change in state of the three vital systems to protect living patients from being treated as dead:

No one shall be declared dead unless respiratory and circulatory systems and the entire brain have been destroyed. Such destruction shall be in accord with universally accepted medical standards.

On July 26, 2023, the first reading of a proposed revision (rUDDA) to the UDDA, the ULC received an overwhelming response in opposition to the recommended changes. The entire proposition has reached a standstill and was tabled thanks to Dr. Byrne's tireless efforts and others sharing convictions like his. A battle was won on this day, but the war is ongoing. Dr. Byrne will not rest until the UDDA is repealed and replaced or until he hears Jesus say: "Well done, good and faithful servant! Enter into the joy of your rest."

Paul A. Byrne: Defender of Life was written to present Dr. Byrne's incredible life and legacy and to inspire many to follow in his footsteps to protect life from conception until death. God created, prepared, and equipped him for this specific end. As one chronicles and studies his life, this testimony about him is revealed page after page in the book. As image bearers of the Creator of life, may we join Dr. Byrne's life's mission by using our unique personalities, experiences, and gifts to oppose the culture of death in America and to defend vulnerable life.

Made in the USA
Monee, IL
01 July 2024